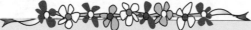

Praises for The Miracle of Fasting and The Bragg Healthy Lifestyle

These are just a few of the thousands of testimonies we receive yearly, praising the Bragg Health Books and *The Miracle of Fasting* book for the rejuvenation benefits they reap – physically, mentally and spiritually. We hope in time to also receive one from you.

When I was a young gymnastics coach at Stanford University, Paul Bragg's words and example inspired me to live a healthy lifestyle. I was 23 then; now I'm over 70, and my own health and fitness serves as a living testimonial to Bragg's wisdom, carried on by Patricia, his dedicated Health Crusading daughter.
Dan Millman, author, *Way of the Peaceful Warrior*
– *www.peacefulwarrior.com,*

Thanks to the Bragg health books, they were our introduction to healthy living. We are very grateful to you and your father.
– Marilyn Diamond, Co-Author, *Fit For Life* – Best Seller – 40 weeks

Paul Bragg saved my life at age 15 when I attended the Bragg Health Crusade in Oakland. I thank the Bragg Healthy Lifestyle for my long, healthy, active life spreading health and fitness.
– Fitness Pioneer, Jack LaLanne, Bragg follower to 96 1/2

The Bragg book *Miracle of Fasting* inspired me to be healthy trim and fit. I gave up all bad habits – smoking, alcohol, swearing. Now I love God. I was an unhealthy 350 lbs. and now a healthy 150 lbs, lean, trim and now I am also a Health Crusader. I've finished 8 Boston Marathons. – Dick Gregory

I give thanks to Health Crusaders Paul Bragg and daughter Patricia for their dedicated years of service spreading health. It's made a difference in my life and millions worldwide.
– Pat Robertson, Host CBN "700" Club

A fast with distilled water can help you heal with greater speed; cleanse your liver, kidneys and colon; purify your blood; help you lose excess weight and bloating; flush out toxins, clear the eyes, tongue, and cleanse the breath. I use your Bragg books for my conversion to the healthy lifestyle.
– James Balch, M.D., co-author, *Prescription for Nutritional Healing*

T0014994

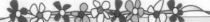

Praises for The Miracle of Fasting and The Bragg Healthy Lifestyle

I've known the wonderful Bragg Health Books for over 25 years. They are a blessing to me and my family and to all who read them to help make this a healthier world. – Pastor Mike Macintosh, Horizon Christian Fellowship, CA

Thanks to Bragg Fasting Book & Healthy Lifestyle, we are healthy, fit and singing better and staying younger than ever! – The Beach Boys • *www.TheBeachBoys.com*

I love the Bragg Health Books and *The Miracle of Fasting*. They are so popular and loved in Russia and the Ukraine. I give thanks for my health and energy. I won the famous Honolulu Marathon with the all–time women's record! – Lyubov Morgunova, Champion Runner, Moscow, Russia

Thank you Patricia for our first meeting in London in 1968. You gave me your Fasting Book – it got me exercising, brisk walking and wisely eating more healthy. You were a blessing God-sent! – Reverend Billy Graham

It was in Hawaii I began to realize that while lifestyle choices can not only be a major negative to health and well-being but lifestyle can be a winning asset to wellness! My discovery on fitness and health began shortly after I arrived in Hawaii at 19 when I discovered fitness and health pioneer Paul Bragg teaching a free exercise class 6 days a week at Waikiki Beach. – Kathy Smith, Hollywood, CA • *www.KathySmith.com*

As a youth I had a learning disability and was told I would never read, write or communicate normally. At 14, I dropped out of school and at 17 ended up in Hawaii surfing. My road to recovery led me to Dr. Paul Bragg who changed my life by giving me one simple affirmation to repeat: "I am a genius and I apply my wisdom." Dr. Bragg inspired me to live a healthy lifestyle and go back to school and get my education and from there miracles happened. I've authored 54 training programs and 14 books and love to health crusade around the world thanks to Bragg. – Dr. John Demartini, Dynamic Crusader • *www.DrDemartini.com*

B

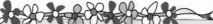

Praises for The Miracle of Fasting and The Bragg Healthy Lifestyle

Thanks to you and your wonderful father for your guidance and teaching over the years. I first read *The Miracle of Fasting* in 1965 after meeting your dad on the beach in Santa Monica in front of my lifeguard tower at Sorrento Beach. I've lost weight, my mind is clearer, my vision has sharpened enough to notice the difference, and I feel closer to my Creator than ever before. Fasting truly is a miracle! What a great gift you and your father have provided for us all through your Bragg health books and wonderful Bragg health products. At 67 years of age I am very thankful for the great benefits of good health I enjoy because of the work you and your father have so generously dedicated your lives to!!! Wishing you every blessing under the Sun. – Captain Wes Herman (retired) Santa Barbara County Fire Department

I've been reading Bragg *Miracle of Fasting* Book since my early days in ministry. I am thankful for all the great Health Crusading that Paul C. Bragg and his daughter Patricia Bragg have done all these years. Thank you for the health books and health products, that are going strong for over 100 years. The Lord loves them and I am thankful for all I have learned from them. – Jentezen Franklin, Pastor, Irvine, CA

Your dad, Dr. Paul Bragg, IS the FATHER of the Natural Health Industry and the entire Natural Health Movement. Everything that has been done in natural health and physical culture since has been based on the pioneering vision and principles articulated by Dr. Paul C. Bragg. He gave us all our direction! – Dr. William Wong, Texas

I bought and have read through the *Miracle of Fasting* ebook twice (plan to read it many more times). I feel so blessed to have found your website, ebooks and Bragg Healthy Lifestyle. I have done two successful 36-hour fasts and now look forward to more, then my first three day fast. I plan to buy all your ebooks within the next week and I love your organic vinegar and amino acids. Thank you so much. – Rick, CA

God promises miracle healings to people who fast & pray. – See Isaiah 58:6-9

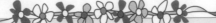

Praises for The Miracle of Fasting and The Bragg Healthy Lifestyle

The Bragg Healthy Lifestyle with Fasting has changed my life! I lost weight and my energy levels went through the roof. I look forward to "Fasting" days. I think better and am a better husband and father. Thank you Patricia, this has been a great blessing in my life. Also, thank you for your sharing The Bragg Healthy Lifestyle at our "AOL" Conference.
– Byron H. Elton, VP Entertainment, Time Warner AOL

Patricia Bragg is a dedicated Health Crusader and she shared her Bragg Healthy Lifestyle with millions of our radio listeners. I have taken the Bragg Organic Apple Cider Vinegar faithfully every day for the last two years. Thank you Patricia.
– Host George Noory, Coast to Coast Radio

Bragg Vinegar and Fasting Books helped me lose 75 lbs. and has increased my regularity and energy. I have the Bragg Vinegar Drink 3 times daily, plus before I sing, it clears the raspiness in my throat. I have acquired a taste for the vinegar and honey mix and love it! It's pretty amazing! – Nonie Hilgesen, Music Teacher, Calvary Chapel Christian School, CA

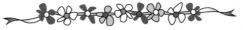

We get letters daily at our Santa Barbara headquarters. We would love to receive testimonials from you on any blessings and healings you've experienced after following The Bragg Healthy Lifestyle with Fasting. It's all within your grasp to be in top health. By following this book, you can reap Super Health and a happy, long, vital life! It's never too late to begin – see (page 91) the study they did even with people in their 80s and 90s and the amazing results that were obtained! You can receive miracles with nutrition, exercise and fasting! Start now!

Daily our prayers & love go out to you, your heart, mind & soul.

Patricia Bragg and *Paul C. Bragg*

D

Patricia Bragg Books

Fasting – Cleanses, Renews and Rejuvenates

THE MIRACLE OF
FASTING

PROVEN THROUGHOUT HISTORY
For Physical, Mental and Spiritual Rejuvenation

PAUL C. BRAGG, N.D., Ph.D.
LIFE EXTENSION SPECIALIST
and
PATRICIA BRAGG
HEALTH CRUSADER & LIFESTYLE EDUCATOR

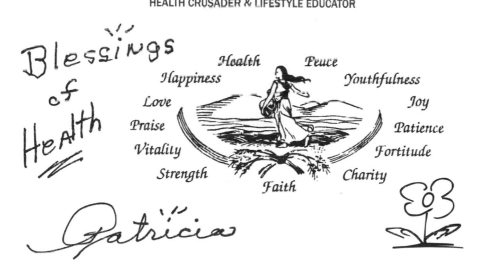

Blessings of Health

Health   Peace
Happiness   Youthfulness
Love   Joy
Praise   Patience
Vitality   Fortitude
Strength   Charity
Faith

Patricia

BECOME
A Health Crusader – for a 100% Healthy World for All!

www.PatriciaBraggBooks.com

The Miracle of
FASTING

Proven Throughout History
For Physical, Mental and Spiritual Rejuvenation

PAUL C. BRAGG, N.D., Ph.D.
LIFE EXTENSION SPECIALIST
and
PATRICIA BRAGG
HEALTH CRUSADER & LIFESTYLE EDUCATOR

Visit our website:
www.PatriciaBraggBooks.com

Fifty-fifth Edition MMXXI
ISBN: 978-0-87790-083-2

Library of Congress Cataloging-in-Publication Data on file with publisher

Published in the United States
HEALTH SCIENCE
7127 Hollister Avenue, Suite 25A, Box 249, Santa Barbara, CA 93117
Toll-Free: (833) 408-1122

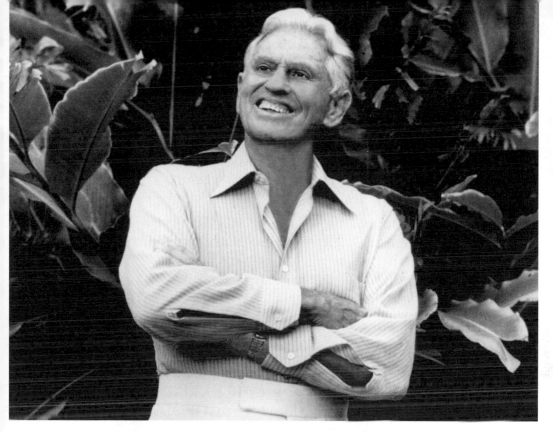

PAUL C. BRAGG, N.D., Ph.D.
World's Leading Healthy Lifestyle Authority

Paul C. Bragg's daughter Patricia and their wonderful, healthy members of the Bragg *Longer Life, Health and Happiness Club* exercised daily on the beautiful Fort DeRussy lawn, at famous Waikiki Beach in Honolulu, Hawaii. On Saturday there were often health lectures on how to live a long, healthy life! The group averaged 50 to 75 per day, depending on the season. From December to March it can go up to 125. Its dedicated leaders carried on the class for over 43 years. Thousands visited the club from around the world and carried the Bragg Health and Fitness Crusade to friends and relatives back home.

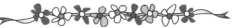

Your body is a non-stop living system, in constant motion 24 hours daily, cleaning, repairing, healing and growing. – Patricia Bragg

To maintain good health, normal weight and increase the good life of radiant health, joy and happiness, the body must be exercised properly (stretching, walking, jogging, biking, swimming, deep breathing, good posture, etc.) and nourished with healthy foods. – Paul C. Bragg, N.D., Ph.D.

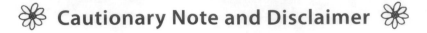

❈ Cautionary Note and Disclaimer ❈

The information provided here is for educational purposes only. Any decision on your part to read, listen and use this information is your personal choice. The information in this book is not meant to be used to diagnose, prescribe or treat any illness. Please discuss any changes you wish to make to your medical treatment with a qualified, licensed health care provider.

If you are taking medication to control your blood sugar or blood pressure, you may need to reduce the dosage if you significantly restrict your carbohydrate intake. This is best done under the care and supervision of an experienced and qualified licensed health care provider. Anyone who has any other serious illness such as cardiovascular disease, cancer, kidney or liver disease needs to exercise caution if making dietary changes. You should consult your physician for guidance. If you are pregnant or lactating, you should not overly restrict protein or fat intake. Also, young children and teens have much more demanding nutrient needs and should NOT have their protein or fat intake overly restricted.

The information presented in this book is in no way intended as medical advice or a substitute for medical counseling. It is intended only to provide the opinions and ideas of the authors. It is sold with the understanding that the authors are not engaged in rendering medical, health or any other kind of professional services in this book. The reader should consult his or her medical doctor, or any other competent professional, before adopting any of the suggestions in this book, or drawing inferences from it.

The authors disclaim any responsibility for any liability, loss or risk, personal or otherwise, which is incurred as a consequence, directly or indirectly, of the use and application of the contents of this book.

Please consult your physician before beginning this program, and use all of the information the authors suggest in conjunction with the guidance and care of your physician. Your physician should be aware of all medical conditions that you may have, as well as medications and supplements you are taking.

Fasting Helps Keep You Healthy and Youthful

Fasting is an effective and safe method of detoxifying the body – a technique that wise men have used for centuries to heal the sick. Fast regularly and help the body heal itself and stay well. Give all of your organs a rest. Fasting can help reverse the ageing process, and if we use it correctly, we will live longer, happier lives. Just three days a month will do it. Each time you complete a fast, you will feel better. Your body will have a chance to heal and rebuild its immune system by regular fasting. You can fight off illness and the degenerative diseases so common in this chemically polluted environment we live in. When you feel a cold or any illness coming on, or are just depressed – it's best to fast!
– James Balch, M.D., co-author, *Prescription for Nutritional Healing*
"Bragg Health Books were my conversion to the healthy way."

v

Forward
By Julia Loggins

Paul Bragg gave America many unprecedented gifts: the keys to reversing illness and disease, lifestyle and dietary practices that have influenced every health enthusiast for the last 100 years; a platform for the importance of organic food, the first health food store, the first health food product company . . . and the toolbox to fasting that has the power to profoundly change your body, your brain and your life.

But the most phenomenal gift he gave us is his daughter, Patricia Bragg. At 92, the message and mission of this icon health evangelist is as potent today as it was half a century ago: that each of us has the power to transform our physical health, our energy, our attitude and our habits to live an extraordinary life. The life Mother Nature intended us to live. To Patricia Bragg, that is a life full of possibilities, free of pain and limitation. It is a life where we are, as she says, the captain of our own ship. And believe me, she is the captain of her ship: uncharted, unsinkable, unstoppable.

Patricia Bragg has spent every day of her adult life not only teaching the principles of health and wellness, but living them. She explains that we "earn our health" through diligent focus on daily rituals, just as we "earn our food" by moving our bodies, and getting our you-know-what off the couch. Everyone who has ever met Patricia Bragg has a story about her, a story that likely entails her telling them - in no uncertain terms – to quit eating junk, get their hands into the dirt and grow their own tomatoes, and to fast, 24 hours a day, once a week. At the very core of the Bragg Program, fasting not only initiates the body's wondrous ability to heal, but fills us with palpable strength and courage. Circling the globe over 30 times, the peerless queen of natural living has taught millions to reclaim their willpower and put down the fork one day a week so that digestion may rest and the soul replenish.

These time-tested teachings saved my life.

When Paul and Patricia Bragg were galvanizing Rachel Carlson into writing the "Silent Spring" – the ground-breaking best-seller that warned America of the dangers of pesticides and chemicals on our food and in our air – I was struggling to breathe in the Intensive Care ward of a hospital in Pasadena, California, home of the Rose Parade, Cal Tech, cheeseburgers and in the 1960's, a thick blanket of smog. I was born in 1955 "allergic to the 20th century," hypersensitive to the chemicals Ms. Carlson wrote about, and suffering from life-threatening asthma, rheumatoid arthritis, allergies and bleeding ulcers. Doctors told my parents I wouldn't live beyond 17. Thanks to the foresight and gumption of a medical doctor inspired by the Bragg principles – who told my parents my only hope was embracing an organic, sugar-free diet – I was able, in time, to throw away my inhaler and dedicate myself to the task of detoxifying a train-load of pharmaceutical drugs, which allowed my organs to regenerate, my gut to shed the scar tissue . . . and my spirit to embrace the awareness that I was put on earth to help others heal, no matter how dire the circumstances or how grim the diagnosis.

Fast forward forty years: There I was, at my table at the Santa Barbara Fermentation Festival, holding my second book, *It Takes Guts to Be Happy!* when Patricia Bragg, in the flesh – flowers in her hair, pink cowboy boots on her feet – bounded over to me, all 4'10" of her. She radiated light and the kind of confidence you can't learn in a self-esteem workshop, (though Lord knows, I had tried). It came from the heart of her, from her core.

She said, "Dear one, do you need some help getting your message out into the world?? I think you do. You know, I can help you!!"

And of course, she did. (Here we are.) And, she can help you. Right here and right now.

Imagine her standing in front of you, glowing with love, not judgement. She doesn't accept excuses; she exudes compassion. Maybe you're feeling a bit shaky, as I was when I met her that first time. No doubt about it, Patricia Bragg can be intimidating,

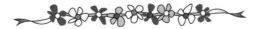

Living in harmony with the Universe is living totally alive,
full of vitality, health, joy, power, love, and abundance
on every level. – Shakti Gawain

something she does not apologize for. She means business. Health is life and she knows it, so why pretend otherwise? She inspires us – demands us – to rise, to pull ourselves together, get in the ring, and not let Mother Nature or our best selves, down.

I understand that you may be sick . . . you may hurt like firecrackers from head to toe . . . and you might not remember if and when you ever felt well. Or, you may be struggling to lose that frustrating fifteen pounds . . . or twenty. Or thirty. Or fifty.

Even more heartbreaking, you may feel as if there is no hope, and maybe every doctor you've seen has told you just that . . . that you won't have that baby you dream of . . . or you fear that the life that flashed in front of you long ago, when you still had a shred of optimism left, was indeed just a dream that would never actualize.

Maybe you've completely lost your faith.

Patricia Bragg would look at you, right into your eyes and say, "Dear, you can do this!! It's never too late. You are going to thrive, and I'm going to teach you how. Read my book and begin by fasting, 24 hours a day, one day a week, and that will start you on the road to health. There is no going back. Today is the day you won the lottery, because your health is your wealth."

Even if you are skeptical, you believe her. Because it's 100% true. And, she would be the first to tell you that she doesn't have all the answers. No one does. When you take charge of your own life, you realize that the only one who knows what is best for you is YOU. This book is your launching pad to tried-and-true information and inspiration that connects you to your inner healer, your Vital Force – the part of each of us that is entirely capable of healing our bodies.

It's not where we stand in the world, but in what direction we are moving.

You are a miracle – self-cleaning, self-repairing, self-healing –
please become aware of "YOU" and be thankful for all your
miracle blessings that take place daily. – Paul C. Bragg, N.D., Ph.D.

The grit and grace of Patricia Bragg – her resolve and her knowing – transcends flesh and time, as does the wisdom of her teachings. As you read her words, step-by-step, we're going to walk this road together. Purification is the foundation of the Bragg Program. Releasing toxins – not only the ones we've ingested and breathed, but all the traumas we've endured and the beliefs that no longer serve us – is where illness ends and your new life begins. If it can work for me, it can work for anyone. Though doctors told me I'd never have children, I have a creative, kind 22-year-old songbird of a daughter and a generous, sharp 27-year-old son, brought up on the Bragg principles. Though our gifts and our life path are unique, we are all health crusaders. The world needs that message now, more than ever.

And the world needs you, too. Whatever your gift is, we need daring, clear-headed, tenacious shape-shifters to heal this sacred planet of ours, and to hold and heal each other.

So buckle up: This IS the best day of your life. The journey may not be for the faint of heart, but the reward is spectacular.

As Patricia Bragg says, "Life is a Miracle."

I'm honored to be here. Let's leap!

~~~~~~

"The greatest discovery by modern man is the method to rejuvenate himself physically, mentally and spiritually by fasting. We can create a quality of agelessness and ignite our body's Vital Force to heal any illness or disease."

Patricia Bragg has spoken – and often shouted – these words hundreds of thousands of times, and does so to this day. These are fighting words, because being healthy is a revolutionary act like no other. When you're healthy, you have wings to fly and the joy of exercising both your muscles and imagination.

When you're sick or in pain, it becomes the focus of your life. I know this first-hand, and I have seen it in my beautiful, brave clients over the last four decades, as they struggle with everything from autoimmune disease to cancer to depression, and innumerable other maladies caused by toxicity and trauma.

I want you to know that sick and diseased is not the new normal. Don't let anyone tell you that. Don't buy it. I didn't; my clients didn't; and millions of Bragg followers didn't.

You have the right to be healthy.

You have the right to be happy.

You have the right to find your purpose in life and soar.

And, no matter how much you love your partner, your children or your dearest friends, if you don't put your oxygen mask on first and heal yourself, nothing else matters. Really.

In healing ourselves, we earn not only a fit, able body, but the kind of self-respect that changes our life, and the lives of those we care most about. Not instantly, but it happens. We are all connected . . . that is Mother Nature's law.

Illness and disease begin with toxicity, and we live in a poisoned world. More than two billion pounds of pesticides are dumped on America's farmlands every year. And, genetically modified foods (GMO's) were designed so they cannot break down or be digested; cancer rates have skyrocketed since their introduction. Believe it or not, we each come into contact with 2500 chemicals a day. These toxins overwhelm our organs of drainage and detoxification, and they are stored in our body and our brain – forever – unless we purify ourselves by cleansing and fasting.

Patricia Bragg writes that, "Autointoxication is the greatest enemy of vibrant health. It's the root cause of all major physical troubles, because illness starts in a poisoned bloodstream. It's the basis of most troubles which affect the heart, liver, kidneys and joints. When our bloodstream and lymphatic system – your river of life – become poisoned, this has more to do with premature ageing than all the other cases combined."

Flushing these toxins is the most effective way to reverse the ageing process and restore the kind of vibrancy that many people haven't experienced since they were ten! As a colon therapist, gut health expert and fasting coach, I have seen this truth in action.

About ten years ago, a colleague sent me a 35-year-old woman whom I will call Mandy. Mandy had been in a mental health facility for two years, and bedridden for a year before that. She barely spoke, her skin was puffy and red; she walked with a limp and was seriously depressed. In fact, she had attempted suicide more than once. My colleague, a medical doctor, said that he could not figure out what to do for her, adding that he would "have my back" if I would be willing to guide her through a cleanse, and see her weekly for colon hydrotherapy. This lovely, now-distraught woman had once been a renowned painter . . . and she painted with oils in a room without ventilation, next to an industrial waste facility that was known to emit dangerous fumes. She had been poisoned without even knowing it.

Our program was simple: One day a week she would fast, gradually building up to two to three fasting days a week, eating as clean as possible in between. (Mandy had no willpower in the beginning, so the process was not a straight line). After three months, her pallor began to shift and her limp lessened. Six months later, she was 25 pounds lighter, entrusting me with stories of her childhood and telling hilarious jokes. In a year, her limp was gone; her mood was steady and eating organic food was her way of life, and she was 50 pounds lighter – her weight as a teenager. All the puffiness had disappeared. If you saw her, you'd never think anything had ever been amiss. She went from dragging to bouncing into my Clinic, cheerful and upbeat as a spring day. That fall, Mandy moved to Maui and is now, happily, painting outside in the sun, under a palm tree. Her paintings hang in my office. She's healed.

I have dozens and dozens of stories like this. They are proof of the invincibility of our Vital Force.

In my book, "It Takes Guts to Be Happy!" I quote some statistics from the World Health Organization (WHO):

- WHO predicts that one in two of us will get cancer
- WHO predicts that one in three Americans will be obese in the next decade
- Autism, in one of its many forms, now strikes one out of 40 children

- Three out of five Americans between 25 and 40 are affected by infertility

- One in four of us are depressed, and half of those are seriously depressed

So many of us are hurting. But we have the power to heal, and to challenge these statistics. We have the power to shift our consciousness and our circumstances by getting to the root of why we are so sick and tired, and doing something about it – something that we can do at home, and that we are in total control of. Our inner healer is always present, even when our minds are overcome with fear – another side effect, ironically, of neurotoxins in our food chain that affects our brain.

In fact, one of the most potent experiences of fasting you will have is the cleansing of your thoughts, which is why fasting has been used by sages and spiritual teachers since the beginning of time. You may discover that as you become comfortable with fasting, you'll turn to it as a tool when confronting a problem, experiencing a change or loss, or looking for an answer to a burning question. You may also want to experiment with a popular form of fasting, called "Intermittent Fasting," which was introduced by Paul and Patricia Bragg. When many Americans were nibbling gooey donuts with sprinkles and sipping coffee with sugar and cream for breakfast, Patricia Bragg was out on the court, playing a fast game of tennis, and diving in to her first meal at lunchtime. In this book, we'll explore Intermittent Fasting, and all the positive implications of cleansing and purification.

Patricia Bragg's wish for you – and mine as well – is for you to wake up as energized and hopeful as Nature intended, and close your eyes at night filled with peace. Fasting is her secret to not only 92 years of radical health and prosperity, but the kind of happiness and joy that most adults rarely possess. We trust with this program, you may be one of them.

Julia Loggins – Santa Barbara, 2020

THE MIRACLE OF FASTING

To preserve health is a moral and religious duty, for health is the basis for all social virtues. We can no longer be as useful when not well. – Dr. Samuel Johnson

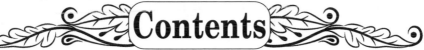

Contents

A good book goes around the world offering itself to reasonable men, who read it with joy and carry it to their neighbors. – Ralph Waldo Emerson

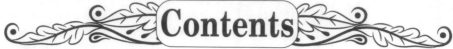

Contents

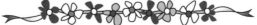

*When you sell a man a book you don't just sell him paper, ink and glue,
you sell him a whole new life! There's heaven and earth in a real book.
The real purpose of books is to inspire the mind into its own thinking.*
– Christopher Morley

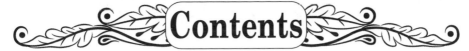

Contents

Knowledge is love and light and vision. – Helen Keller

Contents

Healthy Mind Habits: Wake up and say – "Today I am going to be happier, healthier and wiser in my daily living! I am the captain of my life and I am going to steer it living a 100% healthy lifestyle!" Happy people look younger, are healthier and live longer! – Patricia Bragg

It is never too late to be what you might have been. – George Eliot

Contents

> *"Being optimistic is like a muscle that gets stronger with use.*
> *Makes it easier when tough times arrive. You have to change*
> *the way you think in order to change the way you feel."*
> *– Robin Roberts, Author, "Everybody's Got Something"*
> *and anchor ABC's morning show – "Good Morning America"*

America Needs Volunteers – it's wonderful to be of service – to help
when and where needed. See where you can help others in need:
Websites: VOA.org • OnlineVolunteering.org • VolunteerMatch.org

Kindness should be a frame of mind in which we are alert to every
opportunity: to do, to give, to share and to cheer. – Patricia Bragg

"Eat not for the pleasure thou may find therein;
eat to increase thy strength and health, and eat to preserve
The Life thou has received from Heaven!" – Confucius,
influential philosopher, teacher and political figure, 479-551 BC

Decades of Amazement as Life Rolls By

Where did our years go? They went by so fast.
When we're young they seem to cra-a-wl,
With each decade, they fly past!

At 29 we're the center; At 30 we feel supreme
But 40 strikes terror; Life's not what it seems.
By 50 we've reached maturity; At 60 we accept seniority.
When we're filled with excitement of creative living,
There's no room for depression and despair!

But at 65, wisdom that comes from experience
Then takes over and we learn to accept ourselves as we are.
Each new day is a gift to be treasured,
Enabling us to go far!

At 75, life is for the living
But it is through our sharing, loving and giving
that we reach the Stars of Joy, Peace
and the Possibilities of Eternity!

– by Ruth Lubin, who started writing poetry and sculpturing at 80!
PS: Ruth has been a fan of the Bragg Healthy Lifestyle for over 58 years!

PROMISE YOURSELF . . .

To be so strong that nothing can disturb your peace of mind.

To talk health, happiness and prosperity to every person you meet.

To make all your friends feel that there is something in them.

To look at the sunny side of everything and make your optimism come true.

To think only the best, to work only for the best, and to expect only the best.

To be just as enthusiastic about the success of others as you are about your own.

To forget the mistakes of the past and press on to the greater achievements of the future.

To wear a cheerful countenance at all times and give every living creature you meet a smile.

To give so much time to the improvement of yourself that you have no time to criticize others.

To be too large for worry, too noble for anger, too strong for fear and too happy to permit the presence of trouble.

To think well of yourself and to proclaim this fact to the world, not in loud words but great deeds.

To life in faith that the whole world is on your side so long as you are true to the best that is in you.

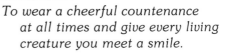

– Christian D. Larson
Author & Influential Leader

Chapter 1

Fasting is the Great Purifier

People are constantly asking and writing us, "Will a fast cure my 'this or that' disease?" We want it clearly and distinctly understood that we are not recommending fasting as a cure for any disease! We don't believe in cures unless Mother Nature and your body do it! We can only inspire you to fast to build more Vital Force to overcome enervation and debilitation. Then as you build your body's Vital Force it will self-cleanse and self-heal.

We recommend that before you begin this program you have a thorough physical examination by an integrative medical practitioner or medical doctor. Have him or her acquaint you with the condition of your heart, arteries and blood. Know your blood pressure, pulse and blood chemistry And then follow this healthy lifestyle for a year and return to your doctor for an exam. We believe your doctor will say you have made a miraculous transformation in your body in one short year. Again, remember, you're only as young as your arteries and miraculous cardiovascular system – your vital river of life.

Your Bloodstream – Your River of Life

Autointoxication is the enemy of vibrant health. It's the root cause of all major physical problems, because illness starts in a poisoned blood stream. It's the basis of most troubles which affect the heart, arteries, liver, kidneys and joints. When your blood stream – your river of life – becomes poisoned, this has more to do with premature ageing than all other causes combined. Keeping your blood pure, clean and healthy is half the battle! The other killer is overloading your stomach and digestive system, giving it a new job before it has finished digesting the last meal.

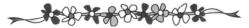

Fasting is the greatest remedy, the physician within.
– Paracelsus, 15th Century Physician, Father of Body Chemistry

The "secret" of the glow of ageless health lies in maintaining internal cleanliness and regeneration. This requires eating natural, organically grown live foods, combined with other healthy practices, such as fasting, drinking distilled, pure water, exercising, and deep breathing. When you purify your body with systematic fasting and live foods, you crave daily exercise. With the knowledge found in these pages, you will find out how you can reap the most out of life, physically, mentally and spiritually.

Bragg Motto – I Love Life & I Want to Live!

At our Bragg Health Crusade lectures, we would often sing our favorite song, *"I Love Life, and I Want to Live"* for students. These strong words express the inner desires to each one of us! **Life in itself is a miracle! And you and I, who have precious life are holding this miracle in the palms of our hands to treasure and protect!**

Fasting Conserves Energy – Your Vital Force

When we fast, we do so on pure distilled water. But when you fast you may add green vegetable juices, clear vegetable broth, herbal teas or if you have low blood sugar, organic bone broth.

Fasting relieves the tremendous amount of digestive stress that eating causes. It takes a huge amount of Vital Force to pass a large meal through the gastrointestinal tract and eliminate the waste via the 30-foot tube that runs from the mouth to the rectum. It's the toxic debris and wastes of metabolism (from the biological process of converting food into living matter and that matter into energy) that brings on so many physical ailments and premature ageing! When the Vital Force of your body drops below normal, then all your physical problems – as well as your mental ones – begin!

Our mental, physical and emotional diets determine our overall energy, health and well-being more than we realize. Every thought and feeling, no matter how big or small, impacts our inner vital force energy reserves.

Fasting is the oldest, fastest and most effective healing method known to man and we are so excited to bring that to you here today.

Chapter 2

Fasting Cleanses, Renews and Rejuvenates

Fasting is the most effective detoxifying method. It's also the safest way to increase elimination of waste buildup and enhance your body's miraculous self-healing, self-repairing process, the one that will keep you healthy and happy for a long life!

Fasting works by self-digestion. During a cleansing fast your body intuitively will decompose and burn only the substances and tissues that are damaged, diseased or unneeded, such as abscesses, tumors, excess fat deposits, excess water and congestive wastes. Even a short fast of one to three days will accelerate elimination from your liver, kidneys, lungs, bloodstream and skin. Sometimes you will experience dramatic changes (cleansing and healing crisis) as accumulated wastes are expelled. With your first fasts you may temporarily have cleansing headaches, fatigue, body odor, bad breath, coated tongue, mouth sores and even diarrhea as you detox and cleanse your body! Please be patient with your body!

3

In this book we will share many practices which will alleviate the discomfort that can come with a cleansing or healing crisis. A cleansing diet for one to two days can greatly facilitate the process of fasting. Fresh salads and organic vegetables, fruits and their juices, as well as fruit smoothies and green drinks (alfalfa, barley green, chlorella, spirulina, wheatgrass) stimulate waste elimination. Fresh foods and juices can literally pick up that dead matter from your body and dispose of it. After a pre-cleansing period, then you can start your fast. Both the prep period and the fast will cleanse your body of excess mucus, old fecal matter, trapped cellular, non-food wastes and they will help remove inorganic mineral deposits and sludge from pipes and joints.

Today begin by eating God's food, drinking plenty of purified water, thinking positive thoughts, affirming aloud, and taking positive action! Then all your tomorrows will become healthier, happier, brighter than you ever dreamed possible! – Patricia Bragg

Daily, even on most fast days, we take 1,000 to 3,000 mgs. of mixed vitamin C powder (a powder that includes acerola, rosehips and bioflavonoids) in liquids. It's a potent antioxidant and helps flush out deadly free radicals. It promotes collagen production for new healthy tissues. It's also important if you are detoxifying from prescription drugs or alcohol overload. **After a fast your body begins to healthfully rebalance when you faithfully follow *The Bragg Healthy Lifestyle*. Your weekly 24-hour fast removes toxins on a regular basis, so they don't accumulate.** Your energy levels will rise and shine – physically, mentally, emotionally and spiritually. Your creativity expands. You will feel like a "new you" – which you are – you are being cleansed, purified and reborn. **Fasting is a miracle!**

Fasting – The Key to Internal Purification

Remember that all these inorganic chemicals must be passed out of your body or they can cause great damage. If the body's Vital Force drops too low then it can't force these inorganic chemicals through your eliminative systems. Then they remain in your body and can cause grave health damage and disease in the future! By fasting we give our bodies a physiological rest. This rest builds our Vital Force and the more Vital Force you have, the more toxins are going to be eliminated from the body each time you fast to keep it clean, pure and healthy.

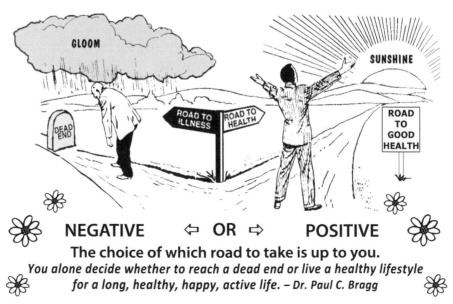

NEGATIVE ⇦ OR ⇨ POSITIVE

The choice of which road to take is up to you.
You alone decide whether to reach a dead end or live a healthy lifestyle for a long, healthy, happy, active life. – Dr. Paul C. Bragg

Chapter 3

Poisons from Chemical Pesticides

All varieties of deadly chemicals are not only sprayed in the air to kill insects, but they are sprayed directly on commercially grown fruits and vegetables. Salads are healthy and appetizing, but often are made deadly because of the use of insecticide sprays. This year's crops have been exposed to more poisonous pesticide chemicals than ever before! Over two billion pounds of pesticides are sprayed on America's farmlands every year. Please be on guard and buy and eat organic non-irradiated produce for your optimal health.

In America deadly DDT was banned due to deaths and health problems! And now these companies sell these poisons to unknowing farmers worldwide – so please beware of foreign fruits and vegetables!

None of us can escape the effects of our current environmental stew that is so challenging for our bodies and minds. In studying brain function, we discovered the breakthrough work of Dr. Michael Merzenich and other cutting edge scientists, who report that our brain is essentially the same one that our distant relatives had in the Stone Age. This explains some of our automatic behavior, such as fight or flight response. Hard-wired responses like this used to be a key to survival in primitive cultures. Today, we rarely need these kinds of safety impulses, and we can learn to manage them, so we are not frying our adrenals and living in a state of constant stress.

Our bodies were originally designed to digest, assimilate, and eliminate the foods that existed thousands of years ago in the natural state they existed, such as: fruits, seeds, nuts, wild greens, and the occasional piece of meat, fish, or eggs. Some would argue that we weren't designed to consume cooked grains, and depending on your ancestors, you may do poorly on dairy products.

A little fasting can really do more for the average sick man than can the best medicines and best doctors. – Mark Twain

The point is, none of our ancestors consumed anything that was processed, sprayed, dyed, preserved, or genetically modified (GMO). Our bodies were not designed to recognize the more than two thousand five hundred foreign substances invented in the last seventy-five years, with which we come into contact every day. The two billion pounds of pesticides that are dumped on America's farmlands each year are foreign agents to our bodies. Genetically modified foods are actually created so they *can't* break down or be digested, and cancer rates have skyrocketed since their introduction.

The Miracle of Fasting Helps Flush Deadly Poisons Out of the Body

6

When we stop eating, which is when we fast, all the Vital Force that has been used to convert food into energy and body tissue is now going to be used to flush all these poisons from our body! When we would travel throughout America and the world lecturing, we were so fortunate to know health-minded people everywhere! We were usually well supplied with organically homegrown fruits and vegetables from their health gardens. But sometimes only commercially grown foods are available, which may have been sprayed with poisonous pesticides. In that case we fast. We faithfully fast to cleanse those toxins out, even when traveling, one 24-hour fast a week!

Fasting – The Miracle Key to Super Energy

Fasting is the miracle key which unlocks Mother Nature's storehouse of energy. It reaches every cell in the body, the inner organs and generates the Life Forces. No one can do it for you! It's a personal duty that only you can perform. No one can eat for you. And we believe that 99% of all human suffering is caused by wrong and unnatural eating. **The efficiency of any machine depends upon the quality and the amount of fuel for generating power it's given. And that goes double for the human machine!**

❀ *Regularly detoxing and fasting will help you cut down the level of harmful chemicals in the body. – Doris J. Rapp, M.D.* ❀

Chapter 4

The Enemy Within Our Bodies

Victor Hugo eloquently called the poison in our body *"the serpent which is in man."* While this remark is poetic, it contains even more truth than poetry. We have come to regard autointoxication (self-poisoning) as the worst enemy in the fight for agelessness and longevity. It is mind-poisoning as well as body-poisoning because, even after the energy of the body is regained, one has a lingering sense of the futility of all other endeavors. Some are inclined to say, *"The best of life is behind me."* *"What lies before is brief and burdensome."* Or *"So many of my friends and relations have gone."* Others say, *"My turn's coming. I've got a date with the undertaker."* These depressing thoughts can generate sad moods and are detrimental to agelessness and longevity! **Remember, we can make the second half of life the best.**

The Bloodstream Should be Alkaline

7

It has taken us many years of research and study to discover the great fact that the bloodstream should be alkaline. Yet, with most of us, it is in an acid state. From headache and indigestion, to pimples and the common cold, most problems arise from acidosis due to self-poisons caused by unhealthy foods! When the life stream is so polluted, how can our immune system defend the body against disease and illness? People unwittingly prepare the body for sickness with their unhealthy lifestyle and then it gets out of control, while they search for a magic pill that will work miracles!

Now if you are as naive as we were, you will ask, *"What can I do to counteract this supposed acidity? How can we cleanse our blood?"* The answer is: *"By supplying it with alkaline-forming healthy foods."*

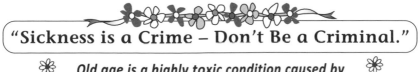

"Sickness is a Crime – Don't Be a Criminal."

Old age is a highly toxic condition caused by nutritional deficiencies and an unhealthy lifestyle!

What Are Alkaline-Forming Foods?

"What are alkaline-forming foods?" People ask us all the time. They are organic, raw fruits and vegetables, salads and leafy greens and lightly steamed vegetables. Three-fifths of your diet should be composed of fruits and vegetables, both raw and cooked. It's always best to enjoy your fresh fruit or a raw vegetable garden salad before you eat any cooked foods.

Alkaline forming foods are the most important to your body. Some of you might say, *"Raw fruits and vegetables will give me gas."* That's because you are on the acidic side and, when you eat the alkaline foods, they start to houseclean and move the toxins out of your bloodstream and body.

Balance Your Alkalinity

Do you know the pH of your body? That is how you measure acidity and alkalinity. Lick or pee on a pH strip and you can find out in two seconds if your pH is out of balance (6.4 to 7.4 is the desired range). Our pH balance is one of the most important chemical balances in our body.

8

An imbalance in the body's pH may lead to:

- Low energy, that "blah" feeling you can't get rid of
- Poor digestion and sluggish elimination
- Hormone imbalances that can lead to infertility
- Depression
- Muscle Cramps
- Headaches and Migraines
- Weight Gain
- Joint Discomfort
- Dry, lifeless skin

And more serious symptoms like:

- Cancer
- Cardiovascular disease
- Bladder and Kidney disease
- Immune system breakdown

Almost every human malady is connected, either by the highway or byway, with the stomach. – Sir Francis Bond Head, 1st Baronet

Gastric acids, such as Hydrochloric acid in the stomach, combine with foods and liquids, and initiate chemical reactions that break down nutrients so they can be digested. Acids are key elements in powering the body. They start up hundreds of organic and chemical processes so we call them the "starters" of life. They are not bad for us and we can't live without them, but they can get out of balance because of our lifestyle.

Electrolytes, The Energy of Life

Electrolyte minerals have the capacity to conduct electricity and they are literally the energy of life. They buffer the acids that these functions create and maintain a perfect acid / alkaline balance, enabling the twenty-two-plus enzymes the body needs to digest food, and to work properly. Without this balance, we are on our way to malnutrition which leads to disease because you are not absorbing any nutrients. We are literally starving! Without this delicate balance, your bowels, alkaline by nature in contrast to the rest of our internal organs, become acidic. And to protect itself, the intestines make a thick mucous barrier inside the colon to guard itself from this acid bath. We call this barrier *"mucoid plaque."*

An acidic pH can create an environment that promotes cancer. When your body doesn't maintain a proper acid / alkaline balance, the cells begin to die. To keep that from happening when there aren't enough electrolytes to buffer digestive acids, the body goes to other parts of itself to find the electrolytes it needs. It will do anything to keep the pH balanced, just like it will do any thing to keep your temperature balanced. That means it will literally cannibalize itself to survive, using electrolyte buffers from your own cells to re-balance you. As a result, your body runs out of these buffers very quickly because so many people eat acidic diets.

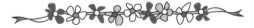

  The accumulation of toxins in the body accelerates ageing.
The elimination of toxins awakens capacity for renewal.
Toxins must be identified and eliminated from your body.
Fasting is Mother Nature's cleansing miracle!

For instance if the body is constantly using the calcium and magnesium that you need to neutralize the acids you consume and burn, when you are in a stressful situation, you become prone to osteoporosis.

When you eat alkaline-forming foods, you have more than enough electrolytes to buffer the acids in your body, provided you aren't eating an overly acidic diet. When you eat acid foods and have stress, which we all do, there are not enough electrolytes to buffer the acids. What is left is an excess of acids and the depletion of electrolytes, which leads to tissue and organ degeneration. Circulation is compromised, and when we have poor circulation, acids accumulate. At a certain point, cancer can develop. With the current statistics about cancer striking one out of two in the population, in the next decade, no one can afford to let that happen.

Keep Your Stomach Healthy and Alkaline

One of the first places electrolytes are compromised is in the stomach. The way to alkalize our bodies is to ingest at least seventy percent alkaline foods until your pH strip measures 6.4.

Because acidosis is more of a negative nature than a positive, we must beware of that. It also affects our mental state. Have you ever said, *"I feel a little blue today, a little low on energy."* Everyone has their off days. But you can maintain yourself in a consistent state of good health, and **honor your body as a fine machine, one that will properly care for you and last a long lifetime.**

At the first suspicion of acidosis, analyze your diet. A grayish tongue, a snappish temper, a flushing of the face; none of these are too trivial! And they are signs of acid. Perhaps today they may not amount to much, but tomorrow they may be more insistent. Acidosis is insidious and accumulative in its action; and it's today, not tomorrow, that we want begin to defend ourself, for life is self-defense! Over-acidity is an adversary that has us at a disadvantage, and what we lack in stamina we must make up for in living a healthy lifestyle!!!

Nothing can bring you peace – but yourself. – Ralph Waldo Emerson

Beware then of acidosis and everything it invites. High-sugar, high-fat and high-protein diets promote acidosis. We must stay away from them and eat a healthy diet rich in fruits, vegetables and grains from healthy organic sources. At the first danger sign, be strong and give up all unhealthy habits and faithfully live *The Bragg Healthy Lifestyle*. This will guide you to super health!

When you live *The Bragg Healthy Lifestyle* you can help activate your own powerful internal defense arsenal and maintain it on guard at top efficiency. Remember that unhealthy eating habits make it harder for your body to fight illness and stay healthy!

Bad Nutrition – #1 Cause of Sickness

"Diet-related diseases account for 68% of all deaths."
– Dr. C. Everett Koop

America's former Surgeon General and our friend, said this in his famous 1988 landmark report on Nutrition and Health in America: *"People don't die of infectious conditions as such, but of malnutrition that allows the germs to get a foothold in sickly bodies!"* Also, bad nutrition is usually the cause of non-infectious, fatal or degenerative conditions. When the body has its full nutrition quota of vitamin and minerals, including potassium, it's almost impossible for germs to get a foothold in a healthy, powerful bloodstream and tissues!

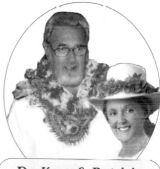

Dr. Koop & Patricia
Hawaii Health Conference

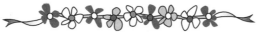

"Paul Bragg did more for the Health of America than any one person I know." – Dr. C. Everett Koop, Former U.S. Surgeon General (1982-1989)

How good it is to be well-fed, healthy and kind, all at the same time.
– Dr. Henry Heimlich, 1920-2016

Knowing and following these teachings will mean true life and good health for you. – Proverbs 4:22

11

Mother Nature Loves You To Enjoy Her Beauty

Let me look upward
into the branches
Of the towering oak
And know that it grew
slowly and well.

Give me, amidst
the confusion
of my day
The calmness of
the everlasting hills.

Let me pause
to look at a flower,
to smell a rose —
God's autograph,
to chat with a friend,
to read a few lines
from a good book.

Break the tensions
of my nerves
With the soothing music
of singing streams
and gentle rains
That live in
my memory.

Follow steps of the godly,
and stay on the right path
to enjoy life to the fullest.
— Proverbs 2:20-21

Mother Nature and friendship are cozy shelters for life's rainy days.

Chapter 5

Fasting Fights Deadly Acid Crystals

Between the moveable joints of every bone in the human body, Mother Nature has placed an abundant supply of a lubricant known as synovial fluid. Take a look at a youngster who is, say 10 years of age, and watch the easy movement of every moveable joint in his body. **Why is this?** I know that your answer would be, *"Well this child is only 10 years of age. I am 66. I can't have the same freedom of movement and the same motion in my joints as a child of 10."* Our answer to you is, *"Why not?"* Years have nothing to do with the amount of synovial fluid that allows the joints to move freely and easily. **There is one main thing that cements your body's moveable joints and that is the build-up of toxic acid crystals.**

Age is not toxic. Just because you're 50, 60, 70, 80 or 90 years old, there should be no diminishing of the vital supply of synovial fluid due to your calendar years.

13

Toxic Crystals First Attack the Feet

There are 26 moveable bones in each foot. The force of gravity sends toxic crystals down into the feet. Gradually feet and ankles start to stiffen, because toxic acid crystals are taking over and replacing the lubrication in the foot joint. Instead of having flexible feet, they become stiff and tire easily. They can ache, burn and cause pain and misery. (Read *Bragg Back & Foot Fitness Program* – see back pages for booklist.) From the feet and ankles, toxic acid crystals and inflammation move upward, causing many to suffer from pains in knees, etc. As time marches on, so does joint deterioration. Soon toxic crystals and inflammation creep into the moveable hip joints. Notice the way people move their hips and how stiff and painful they are.

Few people escape an aching or stiff back. Watch middle-aged people bend over and notice the agony on their faces when they straighten up. Day after day they cry out in anguish, *"Oh, my aching back!"* But the toxic acid crystals and inflammation don't stop in the lower back, they go up the spine, the shoulder blades, the shoulder joints, the neck and elbows . . . eventually creeping into the wrists and fingers. Some people are so full of these toxins that they cannot close their hands or make fists. They all seem to falsely blame one thing: *"I'm getting old."*

Don't believe it. These acid crystals and inflammation are poisons that stayed in your body and cemented themselves in the moveable joints. Billions of pain pills are used by the American public to get relief from their aching joints. Many different medical treatments worldwide are offered to bring relief! **But we are offering you Fasting and *The Bragg Healthy Lifestyle* to guide you onto the road to health so that you can help your body detoxify and heal itself.**

Fasting for Purification

When you fast for 24 to 36 hours, or from 3 to 10 days, the healing power of the body goes to work. This power has always been in your body. This is your Vital Force. When you fast, the Vital Force in your body that would ordinarily be used to masticate, digest, assimilate and eliminate food is then used to purify your body! **That is what fasting is: deep internal cleansing, a physiological rest to build up your body's Vital Force!**

Now, say you have been eating 3 meals a day, whether you were hungry or not, and toxic acid crystals have been deposited into the moveable joints of your body. It's going to take time for Mother Nature and your Vital Force to break down those acid crystals that have accumulated over the years, so please be patient!!!

Fasting is an important part of your program for banishing toxic acid crystals from the moveable joints in your body. You and only you know how free your joints are of this toxic material which causes premature ageing. Start today on your first 24-hour fast. You may be the judge of what effects fasting will have on the many moveable joints of your body. At this very second, roll your head around. Do you hear that grating sound of toxic acid crystals?

We live not upon what we eat, but upon what we digest. – Abernethy

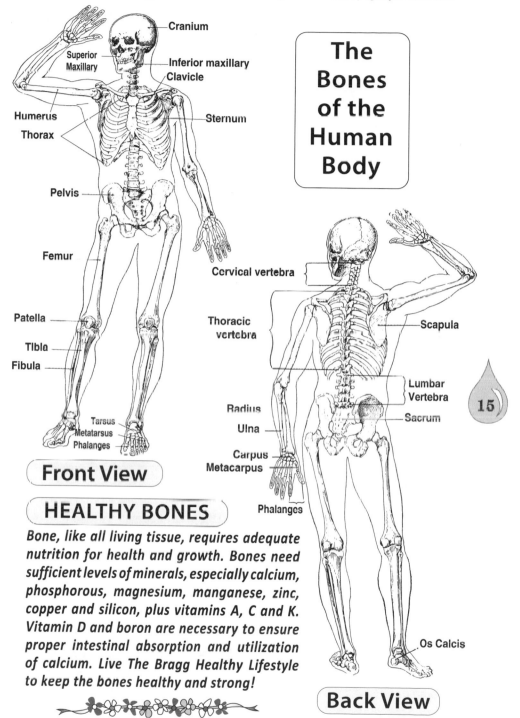

The Bones of the Human Body

Cranium
Superior Maxillary
Inferior maxillary
Clavicle
Humerus
Thorax
Sternum
Pelvis
Femur
Patella
Tibia
Fibula
Tarsus
Metatarsus
Phalanges

Front View

Cervical vertebra
Thoracic vertebra
Scapula
Lumbar Vertebra
Radius
Sacrum
Ulna
Carpus
Metacarpus
Phalanges
Os Calcis

Back View

15

HEALTHY BONES

Bone, like all living tissue, requires adequate nutrition for health and growth. Bones need sufficient levels of minerals, especially calcium, phosphorous, magnesium, manganese, zinc, copper and silicon, plus vitamins A, C and K. Vitamin D and boron are necessary to ensure proper intestinal absorption and utilization of calcium. Live The Bragg Healthy Lifestyle to keep the bones healthy and strong!

Every man is the builder of a temple called his body. We all are our own sculptors and painters, and our material is our own flesh and blood and bones. Any nobleness begins at once to refine a man's features, any meanness or sensuality to degrade them. – Henry David Thoreau

Toxic Acid Crystals Make Joints Grind

The grinding sound you hear is the toxic acid crystals that have deposited themselves on the uppermost bone of your spine – the Atlas. Your fast will not eliminate all the toxic acid crystals from your Atlas, but the bone purification will have started. If you fast one day a week, in one year you will have fasted 52 days. And in that time the Vital Force of your body will have dissolved a large amount of the toxic acid crystals from your joints.

Every time you fast you will notice more freedom in every joint of your body. A feeling of agelessness will replace that tight, stiff, ageing feeling. Once again you will feel free and loose in every moveable joint. You will have Mother Nature, fasting and eating natural foods to thank for your new youthful feeling!

Watermelon and its Seeds are Best Natural Kidney Cleanser . . .

Watermelons are mostly water – about 92% – but this refreshing fruit is soaked with nutrients. Each juicy bite has significant levels of vitamins A, B6 and C, antioxidants, amino acids and lots of lycopene. There's even a modest amount of potassium. Watermelon washes retained poisons and debris out of the bladder without side effects. Always eat melons alone or between meals. It opens your urinary system like a hydrant. Also try watermelon seed tea – 2 tsps ground seeds in quart boiling water, steep, add Stevia sweetener, if desired. Take 3 times daily for fluid retention and kidney cleanser. Sometimes we do 2-3 day watermelon only cleanse, try it – it's great!

Laws of health are inexorable; we see people going down and out in their prime of life because no attention is paid to them! – Paul C. Bragg, N.D., Ph.D.

Vitamins, minerals, herbs and superfoods optimize healing potential. They offer potent armor to deal with the body-ageing realities of today's environment: mineral depleted soil, strong toxic chemical use, and oxygen robbing pollutants. Fortifying your diet with supplements and superfoods strengthens your health and ability to function in a world which makes it tough to be healthy. – Linda Page, N.D., Ph.D., Author of "Healthy Healing"
Visit Doctor Linda Page's website: www.HealthyHealing.com

Yesterday is history. Tomorrow is a mystery. But today is a miracle!!!

Fasting is as Old as Man

The instinct that leads us to fast when the body is sick or wounded resides in the cells of every living being! The reason sick or wounded animals refuse to eat is that is their natural instinct of self-preservation. In this way, the Vital Force (which otherwise would have to be used in the digestion of food) is concentrated at the site of injury to remove any waste products, thus purifying and healing the body. The fasting instinct is so powerful and of such vital importance that, even though semi-civilized man has strayed from the natural path, he is still greatly influenced by this wonderful saving scheme of Mother Nature! If we would only obey the silent voice of this infallible, natural instinct and stop eating when hunger is withdrawn, we would all get well sooner! Better still, we might never get sick again, provided we ate natural food, lived in a natural environment and lived a sane, sensible, healthy, peaceful and natural lifestyle.

Since the infallible intelligence of the living organism withdraws the hunger sensation when there is an excess of food eaten or when the body has been wounded, the wise desire to fast begins when either of those happen.

We read in ancient history that fasting has been practiced since time immemorial by the religious people of the East and by most ancient civilizations! They practiced fasting not only for the recovery of health and preservation of youth, but for spiritual illumination as well. Accordingly, we see the great philosopher, Pythagoras requiring his disciples to undergo a fast of 40 days before they could be initiated into the mysteries of the spiritual teachings. He claimed that only through a 40-day fast could the minds of the disciples be sufficiently purified and clarified to truly understand the profound teachings of the beautiful mysteries of life.

As it was in the old days, fasting will not only purify the body and help restore it to well-being, but has a profound effect on the mental and spiritual parts of men and women.

A full stomach doesn't like to think. – Old Wise German Proverb

Fasting Awakens the Mind and Soul

In our own personal life, as well as the lives of millions of Bragg students who have been conscientious and persistent in their fasting program, great mental and spiritual doors have been opened! If we read a book today, our mind retains what we read as clearly as if the book were right in front of us. Hundreds of our students write that they, too, have developed a keen photographic mind. After a fast of 1 to 3 days, you will notice that a dark cloud has been lifted out of your mind. You can think more logically and can come to decisions quite quickly. What was once a great problem becomes trivial! After a fast, you seem to not get upset and things you worried about are solved more easily by your purified, peaceful, wise mind.

In our personal experience, fasting has helped to develop a keen brain and extrasensory perception. We can find solutions for problems that once caused hours of anxiety and nerve-exhausting worry. Our fasting program has created inner peaceful tranquility of mind. We feel more serene and at peace with ourselves and the world. As you purify your body and mind, you will come closer to a power higher than yourself! This inner strength and inner power, will make you a positive-thinking, youthful person!

The memory becomes sharp as a razor's edge. You can remember names, places and events that go back for years. You will have a better capacity for self-education. Education is not a preparation for life, but education is life itself! To grow mentally and spiritually is the greatest goal we humans can have on this wonderful earth. **Fasting works three ways: You purify your body physically, mentally and spiritually and enjoy more super vitality and health! Your mind becomes a sponge which can absorb new facts and knowledge. Greatest of all are inner peace and spiritual tranquility that make life worth living. Through fasting you will find "Peace of Mind," the greatest and rarest gift of life.**

Periodic fasting keeps you connected to your body's natural tendency to cleanse and rejuvenate. – Pamela Serure, "The 3-Day Energy Fast"

18

Paul C. Bragg Invented Intermittent Fasting by teaching what he calls the "No Heavy Breakfast Plan"

We have taught the "No Heavy Breakfast Plan" to millions of our health followers and readers world-wide. Here's the logical reason why we don't believe in a heavy breakfast. A heavy meal requires most of the nerve energy of the body to handle digestion, thus the mind becomes enervated, making most people dull, sleepy and leaving their precious nerve energy at its lowest ebb!

Let's look at it from another standpoint. Through long years of misinformation, people have been told, *"Breakfast is the most important meal of the day. It gives you the strength, energy and vitality to do a hard morning's work, either physically or mentally."* **This is absolutely erroneous!** It is not a true scientific fact. When you eat a heavy breakfast, through reflex action you feel full and satisfied, but you do not gain strength. It takes hours for this food to be processed by the digestive system before you can gain any energy or vitality. Digestion is a most highly complicated process. Every item of food in the breakfast has to be broken down into fine nutrient fragments so that the body's cells are fed.

19

Morning Resolve To Start Your Day

I will this day live a simple, sincere and serene life; repelling promptly every thought of impurity, discontent, anxiety, fear, and discouragement. I will cultivate health, cheerfulness, happiness, charity and the love of brotherhood; exercising economy in expenditure, generosity in giving, carefulness in conversation and diligence in appointed service. I pledge fidelity to every trust and a childlike faith in God. I will be faithful in those habits of prayer, study, work, nutrition, physical exercise, deep breathing and good posture. I shall fast for a 24-hour period each week, eat only healthy foods and get sufficient sleep each night. I will make every effort to improve myself – physically, mentally, emotionally and spiritually every day.

Morning Prayer used by Patricia Bragg & her father, Paul C. Bragg

---

Dear Friend, I wish above all things that thou may prosper and be in health even as the soul prospers. – 3 John 2

You Must Earn Your Food by Exercising

You can plainly see that healthy eating is a matter of conditioning and habit. We haven't eaten breakfast for years. We woke up early every morning. We hiked, ran, and swam. At our desert home we hiked the hills and rode our bicycles. After several hours of vigorous exercise, we returned home to enjoy our fruit meal and energy drinks. Then we were ready to do our most creative work – we planned the Bragg Health Crusades, wrote articles for health magazines or wrote our books which inspire and guide you to become healthier!

Healthy Eating Habits Keep You Youthful

Around noon we ate our main meal of the day. We started with a delicious salad – see recipes page 125. After salad we had one cooked yellow vegetable – such as baked yam or carrots – one green vegetable, such as Swiss chard, kale, mustard greens, broccoli, zucchini, squash or green beans – and a type of vegetable protein. We enjoyed tofu, beans, lentils and raw unsalted nuts of all kinds and seeds, such as sunflower, pumpkin, and sesame (for Plant Based Protein Chart see page 123).

20

We earned this healthy meal through exercise and activity. Then our bodies were ready to send digestive juices and internal secretions to get full nourishment and energy out of this natural food. The mouth and stomach digestive juices are abundant! Extra benefits included regular exercise, ample fruits and salads which help promote good elimination! This program of 12 meals a week, 2 meals daily, 6 days a week does not burden and exhaust the body's digestive system or the body's bowel eliminative powers (we fasted for 24 to 36 hours a week). On this *Bragg Healthy Lifestyle* program, you don't overeat, and you educate your bowels to move soon upon arising and usually you will have a bowel evacuation within an hour after lunch and sometimes after dinner.

Exercise, along with healthy foods and some fasting helps maintain and when needed restore a healthy physical balance and normal weight for a long, happy, vital life. – Dr. Paul C. Bragg

Juice Fasting is Introductory to Water Fasting

Water Fasting has been rediscovered through Juice Fasting and is a simple and delicious means of cleansing, purifying and rebuilding health and vitality and restoring wellness to the body. To fast is from the Old English word *"fasten or to hold firm."* It's a means to commit oneself to the task of finding inner strength through cleansing of the body, mind and soul. Throughout history the world's greatest church leaders, philosophers and sages including Socrates, Plato, Buddha and Gandhi have enjoyed fasting and preached its many miracle benefits.

Juice Fasts offer people an opportunity to give their intestinal systems rest and cleansing relief from the commercial, high-fat, sugar, salt, protein and "fast food" diets that Americans eat daily.

Many organic raw vegetable juices can be purchased from health foods and juice stores. You can also prepare these healthy juices yourself using a home juicer. It's often best to dilute the juice with $1/3$ distilled or purified water. There are many delicious combinations (see list below) of raw vegetable juices. You may also add nutritious green powders (barley, chlorella, spirulina), and create a powerful health drink even when you are not fasting. When using herbs in these drinks, use 1 to 2 fresh leaves. Seaweed is rich in protein, iodine and iron and is delicious added to fresh vegetable juices.

21

Delicious Juice / Blender Combinations:

1. Beet, celery, alfalfa sprouts
2. Cabbage, celery and apple
3. Cabbage, cucumber, celery, tomato, spinach and basil
4. Tomato, carrot and celery
5. Carrot, celery, watercress, apple, garlic and wheatgrass
6. Grapefruit, orange and lemon
7. Beet, parsley, celery, carrot, mustard greens, cabbage, garlic
8. Beet, celery, kelp and carrot
9. Cucumber, carrot and celery
10. Watercress, apple, cucumber, garlic
11. Asparagus, carrot and celery
12. Carrot, celery, parsley and cabbage, onion, sweet basil
13. Carrot, coconut milk and ginger
14. Carrot, broccoli, lemon, cayenne
15. Carrot, sprouts, kelp, rosemary
16. Apple, carrot, radish, ginger
17. Apple, pineapple and ginger
18. Apple, papaya and grapes
19. Papaya, cranberries and apple
20. Leafy greens, broccoli, apple
21. Grape, apple and blueberries
22. Watermelon (alone is best)

Paul C. Bragg Introduced Juicing to America

Juicing has come a long way since we imported one of the first hand operated vegetable-fruit juicer from Germany. Before this juice was pressed by hand using cheesecloth. Now juices are available to everyone in the American public. TV's famous *Juicemen* – Jay Kordich and Jack LaLanne say that Paul Bragg was their early inspiration and mentor and they both inspired millions to live healthier lives!

Juicers, food processors and blenders are great for preparing foods, drinks, baby foods and diets that are bland. Fibers of juiced fresh fruits and vegetables can be tolerated on most gentle diets. Any raw or cooked fruit or vegetable can be liquefied and added to a broth, a soup or a non-dairy milk. Fresh vegetable juices supercharge your energy and boost your immune system to maximize your body's health power. You may also fortify all of your liquid meals with vegetable powders, such as: alfalfa, barley green, chlorella, spirulina or wheat grass.

The Miracle Life of Ageless Jack LaLanne

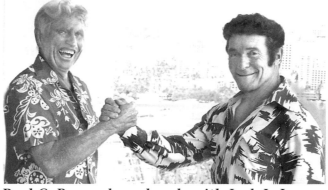

Paul C. Bragg clasps hands with Jack LaLanne

Jack says he would have been dead by 17 if he hadn't attended The Bragg Health Crusade. Jack says, *"Bragg saved my life at age 15, when I attended The Bragg Health Crusade in Oakland, California."* From that day on Jack continued a fulfilled life, living *The Bragg Healthy Lifestyle*, inspiring millions to health, fitness and longevity! – *JackLaLanne.com*

I enjoy eating raw vegetable salads, plenty of organic fruits and fresh juices. I love vegetables, whole-grains, beans, brown rice and lentils.
– See Jack's favorite recipe – Lentil & Brown Rice Casserole on page 125.

Chapter 6

Why We Drink Only Pure, Distilled Water!

Distilled water is pure H_2O – which means it's a compound of 2 parts hydrogen and 1 part oxygen. If you drink rain water, or the fresh juices of vegetables, remember that all of this liquid has been distilled by Mother Nature. If you drink rain water or snow water, there are no inorganic minerals in it. It is 100% mineral-free. If you drink fruit and vegetable juices, you are drinking distilled water plus certain nutrients such as fruit sugars, organic minerals and vitamins. But if you drink lake, river, well or spring water, you are drinking undistilled water, plus the inorganic minerals that the water has picked up. Some of this water is known as hard water, meaning it has high inorganic mineral concentrations that can cause health problems.

There are two kinds of chemicals – inorganic and organic. The inorganic chemicals are inert, which means that they cannot be absorbed into the tissues of the human body.

23

Our bodies are composed of 16 organic minerals which all come from that which is living or was alive. When we eat an apple a day or any other fruit or vegetable, that substance is living. Each has a certain survival time after it has been picked before spoiling. We prefer the vegetarian diet, but the same applies to animal foods, fish, milk, cheese and eggs if you eat them.

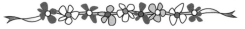

Water flows throughout your body, cleansing and nourishing it. But the wrong kind of water – with inorganic minerals, harmful toxins and contaminants, can clog and gradually turn your body into stone.

❀ *Harmful toxins enter the body through our food, water and air.* ❀

Distilled water is the healthiest and greatest solvent on earth, the only water that can be taken into the body without damage to the tissues.
– Dr. Allen Banik, author of "The Choice is Clear"

Ten Common Sense Reasons Why Distilled Water is Optimal!

- There are over 80,000 toxic chemicals on the market today . . . and 500 are being added yearly! Regardless of where you live, in the city or on the farm, some of these chemicals are getting into your drinking water.

- No one on the face of the earth today knows what effect these chemicals could have upon the human body as they blend into thousands of different combinations. It is like making a mixture of colors; one drop could change the color.

- The equipment hasn't been designed to detect some of these chemicals and may not be for many years to come.

- The body is made up of 75% water (shown on page 74). Therefore, don't you think you should be particular about the type of water you drink to maintain the health of your miracle body?

- Navy Officers / Sailors have been drinking distilled water for years!

- Distilled water is chemical and mineral free. Distillation removes all the chemicals and impurities from water that are possible to remove. If distillation doesn't remove them, there is no known method that will.

- The body does need minerals . . . but it is not necessary that they come from water. There is not one mineral in water which cannot be found more abundantly in food! Water is the most unreliable source of minerals because it varies from one area to another. The food we eat – not the water we drink – is the best source of organic minerals!

- Distilled water is used for intravenous feeding, inhalation therapy, prescriptions, baby formulas and kidney dialysis. Therefore, doesn't it make common sense that it is good for everyone?

- Thousands of water distillers have been sold throughout the United States and around the world to individuals, families, dentists, doctors, hospitals, nursing homes and government agencies. These and other informed, alert consumers are helping protect their health by using only pure, distilled water. Be health wise – do the same.

- With all of the toxic chemicals, pollutants and other impurities in our water, it only makes good common sense you should clean up the water you drink Mother Nature's wise, inexpensive way through distillation!

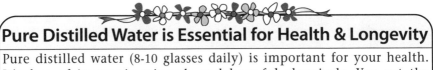

Pure Distilled Water is Essential for Health & Longevity

Pure distilled water (8-10 glasses daily) is important for your health. It's free of inorganic minerals and harmful chemicals. You get the organic minerals you need from your healthy foods. Please read the Bragg Book: *"Water – The Shocking Truth."* Water is key to all body functions: heart, circulation, digestion, bones, joints, muscles, metabolism, assimilation, elimination, glands, sex, energy and nerves.

For more info on water read pages 67-74.

Millions Drink Rain (Distilled) Pure Water!

By drinking distilled water, you will be joining the millions worldwide who drink unpolluted rain water. Man evolved drinking rain water. In Bermuda, where soil is so porous that water cannot be held in the soil, people have special roofs to catch rain water so that it drains into tanks under their houses or nearby.

Distilled Water is Best for Your Health

Years ago, during an expedition to the Atlas mountains of Morocco, we found vigorous people roaming the desert, and the only water they drank was unpolluted rain water.

Every liquid prescription that is compounded in any drug store the world over is prepared with distilled water. It is not true that distilled water leaches the organic minerals out of the body, nor is it dead water. It is the purest and safest water that we can drink!

Distilled water also helps to dissolve the toxic poisons that collect in people's bodies. It passes through the kidneys without leaving inorganic pebbles and stones. If you wash your hair in distilled water you will discover the softness of this naturally soft water.

25

No new water has been created on the face of the earth since it was originally formed. Just as the same energy is formed and reformed, so is the same water used and re-used over and over again by the miracle of Mother Nature. Waters of the earth are purified by natural distillation. The sun evaporates the water. It is collected into clouds and the clouds become full and then we have rain and dew . . . perfectly clean water, one of Mother Nature's great miracles! Who dares to say that they supply man with dead water! **Distilled water is the purest water on earth and it's free of all harmful inorganic minerals and toxic substances.**

We predicted that some day man would need clean, pure water so desperately that great government distillation plants would have to be installed at the seas to convert the unlimited supply of salt water into pure water for all purposes. We have lived to see our prediction come true. Even in Santa Barbara, California they had to build a plant during a long dry spell.

Great Benefits From Short and Long Fasts

Let us again state emphatically that fasting is a science. Please do not force yourself into a long fast because you think the long fast is going to do wonders, unless you are under the strict supervision of a health expert. And even the expert may decide that you would benefit more from shorter fasts to first condition yourself to a longer fast. Your 24-to 36-hour weekly fast, and your 3-to 4-day fasts will provide you with the fasting experience you will need should you wish to try a longer fast later.

We have found in our research on fasting that even the health experts disagree on how long one should fast to get optimal results. Health opinions worldwide vary on fasting lengths from 7 to 30 days. We personally don't believe in longer fasts unless it is really an emergency – and then it is imperative that it be supervised by a health expert or your doctor. **We have millions of students worldwide following this fasting program that we are presenting to you in this book. They are delighted and satisfied with the marvelous health benefits that they enjoy! And we are sure that you will too!!!**

Fasting Is Appreciated Worldwide

The German fasting resorts believe the ideal fast is 21 days. The French are in favor of not more than a 14-day fast. In England they feel a 30-day fast is best. In our American fasting resorts, many fasts are supervised from 14 to 30 days. We have found that in foreign and American fasting resorts, the directors are dedicated people who have a thorough knowledge of fasting. And they have all been successful with people with many complicated physical problems!

Fasting is a great and wonderful science and there is so much to learn about it. We've been supervising fasts for over 80 years. During these fasts we have faithfully fasted and enjoyed wonderful benefits! It is our honest opinion that if anyone fasts over 10 days they should be under the guidance of a health expert.

We believe that the average person can faithfully fast 10 days without any complications. The 10-day fast results in a great amount of internal housecleaning. We sincerely hope that we are not putting any fearful thoughts in your mind about the great science of fasting. There are thousands of people worldwide who supervise their own fasts and some even fast 20 to 30 days. When we spoke on fasting at the Bragg Health Crusades worldwide, we asked our students how many have supervised their own fasts. We have found that thousands of Bragg followers have fasted 20 or 30 days or more with great results and no problems!

But, we still feel that if you do a longer fast, it's wise to be under the guidance of a health expert or doctor, who knows how to control those fasts and knows what is going on with your body. They will be ready to help when toxic poisons are being eliminated and they may advise you to break the fast, because they feel that you have loosened enough toxic poisons for this particular fast. **Always be flexible, kind and loving to your precious miraculous body and never hesitate to reach out to a health expert for guidance!**

Short Fasts Need Good Nutrition and Good Healthy Lifestyle Habits Between Fasts

We know that the wheels of progress grind slowly, but surely. Here is our theory on the science of fasting. We're dealing with human nature and there are many fears in each of us. We believe that people will experiment with the science of fasting if they do short fasts. Many people are willing to try a 24-or 36-hour fast and, when they find that they feel better and look better, they will then attempt a 3-day fast because they have confidence. The next thing you know, they will fast successfully for 7 to 10 days. Many of our students who took several 10-day fasts had such good results that they tried a 15-day fast. And some even went on to 21 days and others tried the full 30 days by themselves.

After fasting, your body becomes cleaner, stronger and full of energy. Remember it's pollutants in the body that cause sluggishness.

27

But they wisely started with the 24-hour fast and then graduated to the longer fast. The more experience and good results you gain, the stronger belief you will have in fasting. If you have never fasted before, start with a 24- to 36-hour fast weekly. We urge you to be the judge of the wonder-working miracle powers of fasting.

Then you may graduate to the 3-to 4-day fast and, after that, a 7-to 10-day fast that will make you feel so proud of your willpower. You can accomplish a great amount of internal cleansing on short fasts. Remember, it's cumulative. The more you fast, the cleaner you become inside. Just make sure that between fasts you are faithfully living *The Bragg Healthy Lifestyle!*

Pre-Cleanse Diet Brings Better Fasting Results

If you prepare for a fast by eating a cleansing diet for 1 to 2 days, this can greatly facilitate the cleansing process. Fresh varieties of salads, vegetables and fruits and their juices, as well as green drinks (alfalfa, barley, chlorophyll, chlorella, spirulina, and wheatgrass) stimulate waste elimination. Live, fresh organic foods and juices literally pick up dead matter from your body and carry it away. Follow this pre-cleansing diet for a few days, and then you will be prepared and you can start your liquid fast.

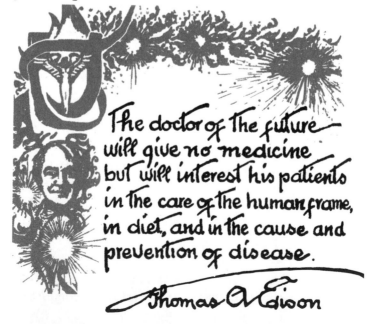

The doctor of the future will give no medicine but will interest his patients in the care of the human frame, in diet, and in the cause and prevention of disease.

Thomas A. Edison

28

Chapter 7

How to Break a 24-Hour Fast

Your 24-hour fast can be from lunch to lunch or from dinner to dinner, as long as you abstain from solid food. This is known as a juice or water fast.

One exception to the 24-hour fast is to add 1-2 Tbsps. of organic, raw, unfiltered apple cider vinegar or fresh lemon juice to 3 of your 8 to 10 glasses of water. You may also add a teaspoon of honey or 100% maple syrup to taste, or if you are a diabetic or have low blood sugar you can use Monk Fruit or Stevia. This drink acts as a mucus and toxin desolver, plus makes the water more palatable. This helps flush debris out through the kidneys. They play a vital part in your fast. This is why it's important during any fast to drink 8 to 10 glasses of pure distilled water.

Your Kidneys – The Miracle Organs

Just think of it – each of the 2 kidneys in your body have a million efficient filters. When the body is fasting, the kidneys step up their work of detoxification. All of the Vital Force and nervous energy of the body is now working overtime to cleanse and heal your body, because it's not being used up in the laborious task of mastication, digestion, metabolism and elimination. You have no idea how powerful the Vital Force is in your body until you experience this great fasting body renovation!

That experience will mark a new day in your entire physical structure. That is the day you will start to understand what superior health means! Your Vital Force will increase so greatly with each fast. You will purify your kidneys and all your other organs.

By relieving your body's work of digesting foods, fasting allows your system to rid itself of toxins while facilitating healing! Fasting regularly gives organs a rest and helps reverse the ageing process for a longer and healthier life. Bragg Books were my conversion to the healthy way. – James Balch, M.D., co-author, "Prescription for Nutritional Healing"

Keep Your Spirits and Morale High

Please understand, even when you take a 1-day fast you are cleansing and purifying your whole body. The very thought that you are building a painless, tireless and ageless body will be your incentive to keep your morale high during your fast.

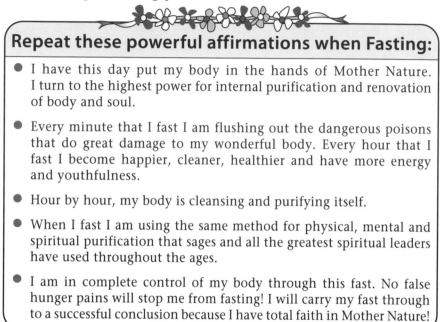

Repeat these powerful affirmations when Fasting:

- I have this day put my body in the hands of Mother Nature. I turn to the highest power for internal purification and renovation of body and soul.

- Every minute that I fast I am flushing out the dangerous poisons that do great damage to my wonderful body. Every hour that I fast I become happier, cleaner, healthier and have more energy and youthfulness.

- Hour by hour, my body is cleansing and purifying itself.

- When I fast I am using the same method for physical, mental and spiritual purification that sages and all the greatest spiritual leaders have used throughout the ages.

- I am in complete control of my body through this fast. No false hunger pains will stop me from fasting! I will carry my fast through to a successful conclusion because I have total faith in Mother Nature!

Just remember, you must give instructions to all the body cells with your total mind (your computer) and your heart. The thoughts you send to your body are going to be carried out by your cells. That is the reason we urge you not to discuss your fasting program with relatives or friends who may not understand. They may give you a negative reaction. Fasting is a personal matter. Keep it that way!

When the toxins are passing out of your body and you feel some discomfort, just say to yourself . . . *"This too will pass."* When we are strong-minded, wonderful results occur. Rejoice that you have been led to this great easy-to-do natural cleansing and rejuvenation miracle.

Wherever you go, no matter what the weather,
always bring your own sunshine. – Anthony J. D'Angelo

Don't Worry About Bowels During the Fast

One of the great worries that most people have who fast is that their bowels will stop moving. It's important for your bowels to move daily. So you may do enemas or colonics to assist your body in flushing toxins. Colon cleansing is thousands of years old. It's written about in the *Essene Gospel of Peace* and the *Dead Sea Scrolls*. Colon Therapies have been a fundamental part of traditional yoga practices, as well as Taoist training. Hippocrates himself, recognized as one of the founders of western medicine, practiced and prescribed enemas for his patients.

When your fast is over and you are again eating well-balanced foods that are high in bulk, moisture, lubrication, and you are drinking 8 glasses of distilled water, your bowels will begin to move again. Try to eat 60% - 70% raw foods in the form of organic salads, sprouts, fruits, veggies and their fresh juices. Faithfully living *The Bragg Healthy Lifestyle* promotes a healthier colon and regular elimination.

31

Decades ago we introduced flaxseeds to the American public and millions have benefitted from them. You can grind 3 Tbsps of flaxseeds and sprinkle them in foods, smoothies, etc. Flaxseeds are nature's richest source of Omega-3 for your heart health. They help repair cells and tissues, transport oxygen, satisfy hunger and help burn up excess body fat. Paul Bragg invented the *Flaxseed Tea Cleanse* (see below). This can be drunk hot or cold.

Flaxseed Tea Cleanse – Drink it Cold or Hot

Mix 1 tsp. ground flaxseed in 8 oz. of water. For hot tea boil 8 oz. of water with 2 tsps. flaxseeds for 2-3 minutes. Let sit another 3 minutes and strain while still hot and drink. Take 3 times per day.

This is an excellent colon cleanse and will not add fiber to your diet during your cleanse. It is also non-inflammatory and gentle for even sensitive colons.

Everyone has a doctor within himself. We just have to help it in its work.
The natural healing force within each one of us is the greatest force
in getting well! – Hippocrates, Father of Medicine, 400 B.C.

The Body Can Take a Lot of Abuse!

The average person believes that if they have one good bowel movement a day, usually in the morning, they are free of constipation. Not so – one full bowel movement a day is not sufficient to remove all food material the average person stuffs into their intestinal tract. As a consequence this rotten, putrefying, morbid, toxic waste lies in the intestine, where it undergoes bacteriological changes that can cause severe health problems. In the United States this caused a million colon cancer cases alone.

The human body is inherently strong and can take a lot of abuse. It is most difficult to tell people who eat incorrectly and have only one bowel movement a day that they are actually constipated and are inviting serious troubles. But there is one warning signal – an unhealthy tongue – that can tell anyone that they are carrying a nasty cesspool within their bodies.

If everyone could fast 2 or 3 days on distilled water, their "Magic Mirror" tongue (page 35) would tell them plainly that they are carrying a horrible mass of fermenting poison inside their intestines. A few days of fasting will coat the tongue with a thick, white, toxic material that has a strong odor if the person is toxic. This whitish coating can be scraped off and examined. In fact, you can spoon-scrape and brush the tongue clean but, in a few hours, the coating returns. This is an indication of the amount of putrefying toxic filth, mucus and poisons that are accumulated in the body's cells that are now being eliminated from the inside surface of the stomach, intestines, organs and from all parts of the entire body. **This is one of the miracles of fasting.**

The actual amount of toxic material that the average person carries around in their intestine is almost unbelievable! Anywhere from 5 to 25 pounds. In my opinion, many physical problems are the result of this clogging of the 30-foot intestinal tube, the cells and the entire circulation of the human body, especially plugging up the microscopically tiny blood capillaries.

The toxic poisons generated by overeating or eating too many of the wrong foods, can damage one of the body's most important organs – the liver. Few people realize how important their liver is to life. It's a great chemical laboratory with many functions. It not only gives forth bile, but it is the body's greatest garbage disposal.

The liver and intestines are partners in this digestive process! If one is sick, the other comes to its aid until it too, breaks down. When the liver and digestive systems break down you're in serious trouble! That's why you often find a sensitive swollen liver, a pasty complexion and jaundice and chronic fatigue, with ongoing constipation.

Important Parts of the Digestive System

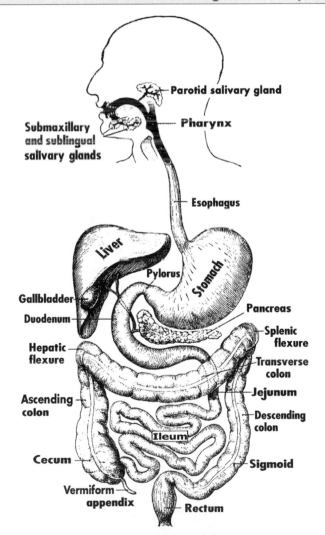

Give Your Vital Force a Chance to Clean House!

So it's plain that when you stop eating to give your body's Vital Force a chance to clean house . . . you will miss the food habit the first few days of your fast! It can be uncomfortable when we allow it! Think positive!

When you fast, your Vital Force loosens the waste in your body and gathers it up to be discarded. As long as this goes on you might feel some discomfort. Colonics and enemas, can ease that discomfort. But once the waste is discarded through the kidneys, you will begin to feel better. We also recommend saunas and dry brushing (see page 132).

As you fast, conditions change from day to day. When your body is eliminating heavy amounts of toxic poisons through the kidneys and other organs of elimination, you might feel some discomfort. But it should also be clear that when you feel better on the seventh day of a ten day fast, better than you did on the third day, that you are improving. Many of the toxic poisons that gave you trouble have been already flushed out! Many people who fast under our supervision feel better and stronger on the tenth day of the fast than they did on their very first day.

34

Good Elimination is Important For Health

It's natural to squat to have bowel movements. It opens up the anal area more directly. When on the toilet, put your feet up 6 to 10 inches on a waste basket or a footstool and that will give the squatting effect. Now raise your arms, stretch your hands above your head so the transverse colon can push to empty out with ease. It's important for you to always drink 8 to 10 glasses of water a day! Enemas and colonics can assist your fast and ease any discomfort that you have.

Fasting is your body's miracle "house cleaning" that focuses on removals, repairs and building of new cells! – Jason Fung, M.D.

Fasts are vitally important – they give the body a break from the digestive process and allows the body to release stored toxins and flush them out!

Learn to Read Your Tongue's Message

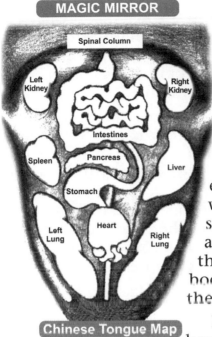

MAGIC MIRROR

Spinal Column

Left Kidney

Right Kidney

Intestines

Spleen

Pancreas

Liver

Stomach

Left Lung

Heart

Right Lung

Chinese Tongue Map

Mother Nature shows by a coated tongue that the body contains toxic poisons. Characteristics of the tissue construction of the powerful internal organs – kidneys, liver and all the glands – are like a sponge. Doctors of the *olden times* always looked at tongues before an exam. Imagine a sponge filled with thick paste. We have supervised millions of fasts and seen huge amounts of the toxins people store in their body while trying to survive on the Standard American Diet.

During a cold, stop and think how much mucus and phlegm passes out of the body through the nose and throat? This is also how the vital organs, such as the lungs, kidneys and bladder pass out poisons during this cleansing fast or cleansing crisis.

Now start to learn about yourself by fasting and watching your tongue, the spongy organ whose surface accurately mirrors the health or ill health of every other part of your body. **The "Magic Mirror" can be a guiding star in your journey to Super Health.** The more faithfully you follow a good fasting and natural eating program, the cleaner your tongue will become during a fast. Also daily when you brush your teeth, brush or spoon scrape your tongue from the back to the tip.

This is definitely a signpost that you are on your *New Bragg Healthy Lifestyle Road* – a life free of physical problems and misery. This road will lead you to your greatest achievement – an Ageless, Painless and Tireless Body! As you go on your 24-to 36-hour fast or your 7-to 10-day fast, note how much cleaner and cleaner your tongue will become. This will reveal the amazing Miracles of Fasting to you!

Daily Tongue Brushing is a Good Habit

You should cleanse your tongue by gently scraping its surface with a spoon's round tip. Begin at the back of tongue and press down and pull spoon forward towards your tongue's tip; repeat as necessary until the entire top of the tongue has been cleaned of its toxic coating. The toxins scraped show one of your immediate *fast* results.

After scraping your tongue, use your toothbrush to lightly brush your tongue from back to tip. Then you can gargle with a mixture of 1 tsp of organic apple cider vinegar in half a glass of water to rinse any remaining germs or toxins from your mouth. Repeat this cleansing 1-2 times daily during a detox water fast or a beginner's juice fast. Your body will continue to push toxic slime out the tongue! This tongue coating shows you that you are doing deep cleansing. It's an accurate indication of the amount of decaying filth, rotting mucus and other poisons that are stored in the tissues that are now being eliminated from the inside surfaces of the stomach, intestines and your entire body.

Fasting Helps Keep The Body Clean & Healthy

We do not die of old age! It's been proven that there are no special diseases due simply to old age. Most diseases kill both young and old. And many diseases start from a body loaded with toxic poisons. Keep the body clean by following your regular fasting program, and eating only healthy foods. Your tongue will be a guidepost to internal purity. Watch it when you do a cleansing fast and see results.

Oil Pulling May Transform Your Health

An Ancient Ayurvedic remedy for oral health and detoxification is oil pulling! It involves use of a pure oil – such as organic coconut oil, for pulling harmful bacteria, fungus and other organisms out of the mouth, teeth, gums and even the throat. All you need to do is place about a tablespoon of oil into your mouth and swish it around for about 10-15 minutes, then spit it out, DO NOT swallow! Lipids in the oil pulls out toxins and the oil absorbs toxins and bacteria. The oil helps in cellular restructuring, proper functioning of lymph nodes and other internal organs. – *OilPulling.com*

Chapter 8

Fasting 7 to 10 Days, Four Times a Year

Our Bragg fasting program calls for four longer fasts a year, along with weekly 24-hour to 36-hour fasts. Fasting helps cleanse and keep your body healthy. These cleansing fasts will help you live a longer, healthier and more vital life! So, our calendar calls for an early January fast. Sometimes this lasts 7 days, it may run 8, 9 and sometimes it may extend the full 10 days.

At the beginning of each year we mark the days we are going to fast for 7 to 10 days. You may wonder why we say "7 to 10" days. Sometimes we fast only 7 because we feel that in that time we have accomplished the necessary body "house cleansing." Be flexible on a date if you feel a cold coming on. Colds call for an earlier start date to your fast to help cleanse the mucus toxins. Colds indicate your body needs detoxifying and a good cleansing. A cold is Mother Nature asking you to fast!!!

37

Fasting Balances Your Thermostat Naturally

We have fasted for so many years that we are perceptive to what a fast is doing for us. Our inner voice seems to tell us when it's time to break a fast. **Remember, let your body and your inner voice guide you, for your body wants you to be healthy, alive and have all the toxins removed!**

We mark our calendar for a fast in the spring, fall, winter, and summer. Our spring fast always runs the full 10 days because that is when we truly want to "clean house" after a long winter. During our Bragg Health Crusades, we were often forced to talk in over-heated halls and auditoriums. We were sorry to say that many people cannot take the cold weather, nor can they stand a fresh, healthy, well-ventilated hall. So we would forget our feelings and lecture in these over-heated halls to the hot-house plants of modern civilization that so many people have become.

Fasting greatly purifies the body and exhilarates the body's functions so the thermostatic system of the body works with efficiency. For instance, we could leave our desert home near Palm Springs, California, in January – when the heat averages in the 80s during the day and in the 60s at night – board an airplane to Midwestern cities such as Duluth or Minneapolis, or a Canadian city such as Toronto – where the temperature would be as low as 10 to 30 degrees below zero and, because of fasting and natural living, our bodies would adjust to this bitterly cold winter weather.

We find that we can take frigid weather better than most of the inhabitants who are supposedly acclimated to their own climate. This ability to adjust to climate is just one of the many fasting miracles that happen to the body. Fasting gives the body a chance to flush out the toxic poisons and build up its Vital Nerve Force.

When summer rolls around, we take a 7-day fast in late July or August. And this is the easiest of all of our fasts because we have been eating large amounts of luscious, organic fresh fruits and garden-fresh organically grown vegetables. We believe that we enjoy our summer fast more than any other. This fast is so easy that we never stop our heavy physical exercise or mental activities. The autumn fast can be anytime in late October or during November. It also extends from 7 to 10 days.

Fasting truly has many cumulative miraculous effects. We fast 75 or more days a year. It's a great physiological rest that we give our bodies and digestive organs! This includes our liver, gallbladder, and all other faithful organs, including ones producing hormones, that run our body and keep us healthy! The physiological rest we give our pancreas allows it to produce ample insulin. This also goes for the stomach, where so many digestive juices are needed to handle and digest food intake.

Mother Nature Intended the Body and Breath to Be Sweet and Free from Odors

You will find that after a fast you'll have more saliva which contains the important enzyme amylase. You will discover that your mouth will taste sweeter and your breath will be clean. The more you fast, the less mouth and body odor you will have! We have never needed deodorant!

Several years ago we supervised a fasting program for a student who came to California from New York. His problem was a terrifically bad body odor that exuded from every part of his body, particularly from under his arms, the palms of his hands and his feet! The odor can only be described as putrid. It wasn't that the man didn't take baths – he took as many as 3 or 4 hot, soapy showers or baths a day and he would use all kinds of deodorants and antiperspirants. But it was to no avail. He was a nervous wreck. He not only had a bad body odor, but heavy halitosis (which is bad breath) and it could just knock you over! He used gargles, lozenges, mint mouth sprays, but he still had rancid, bad breath.

When questioning this man before putting him on his fast, we found that he had been enervated by poor lifestyle habits, overwork, marital difficulties and heavy financial responsibilities. When you enervate yourself, over-extend your nervous energy and exhaust your Vital Force, the elimination organs can't do their job effectively and efficiently. This man was plainly suffering from chronic nervous fatigue! His eating habits were unhealthy. His work day was so busy that he would gobble a sandwich and wash it down with coffee. He didn't take time to prepare healthy meals. He was constipated and his elimination was off its rhythm.

No man can violate Nature's Laws and escape her penalties! – Julian Johnson

Health is the most natural thing in the world. It is natural to be healthy because we are a part of Mother Nature – we are nature. Nature is trying hard to keep us well, because she needs us in her business.
– Elbert Hubbard, American writer, publisher, artist, and philosopher

39

We told him that it took him years to get his body into this decaying condition and a program of fasting and natural living would take time to accomplish its mission of health and wellness. But he was an intelligent and logically thinking man and fully cooperated with *The Bragg Healthy Lifestyle* Program. We started him on a series of 36-hour fasts and between fasts, we added more raw organic fruit and vegetables to his heavily concentrated diet of refined sugars, fats and meat. We believe that there must be a transition period between changing from an unhealthy diet to a healthy diet. It's best not to force the change overnight. Take things slowly. Instead of eating meat three times a day, now he ate it 3 times a week. He had been eating white bread before, so we substituted 100% whole grain bread. His hard work and dedication following *The Bragg Healthy Lifestyle* had him smelling good and feeling healthy from the inside out.

The Ideal Elimination Program

In our life, by living on a diet which is rich in bulk, moisture, water and lubrication, we have established the following good elimination habits. We have bowel movements shortly after arising. We encourage this by a few waist twists and leg kicks to help us achieve a good elimination. We don't eat breakfast because we believe the *No Heavy Breakfast Plan* is healthier. Several hours after arising, we then eat delicious fresh fruits or a dish of fresh sliced organic pineapple, banana, orange, papaya, or a Bragg Energy Smoothie (page 124), a dish of prunes or sundried apricots pre-soaked in pineapple juice. At noon we have our first real meal of the day, a Raw Vegetable Salad (page 125). We often add delicious avocado and additional fresh organic veggies which are excellent lubricants promoting healthy elimination.

We make it a hard and fast rule to always eat salad first. We believe that we are educating our 2,000-8,000 taste buds to accept only natural foods. Therefore when you have raw organic foods, either a raw organic vegetable salad or fruit salad first to start the meal, you are educating your taste buds to enjoy and want fresh, live, healthy foods!

Most people start a meal with a broth or soup and then sandwiches or bread. In our opinion this is wrong! To keep the taste buds keen, sharp and alive – have your fresh raw salad or fresh fruits first, that will start the digestive juices flowing for raw foods which are rich in natural healthy enzymes! This habit contributes to good nutrition! We urge you to always eat something raw at the beginning of each meal. You will find in time your taste buds will begin to reject devitalized, unhealthy foods that you used to be tempted to eat! As you re-educate the taste buds to enjoy fruits and salads, you will find that you can and should increase the daily amount of raw, live foods you eat to 60% of your total intake – that's the healthiest!

The Bragg Healthy Lifestyle Promotes Super Health & Longevity

Remember that raw organic foods are the live, vital foods. They are as Mother Nature made them. They're whole, natural, live foods – vibrating with enzymes and solar energy! Most people want food that stimulates them – sugars, fats, salt, heavy, overcooked and refined foods that have little food value. They want fast foods and most of those have been stripped of their health goodness.

41

The Bragg Healthy Lifestyle consists of eating 60% to 70% fresh, live, organically grown foods: raw vegetables, salads, fresh fruits and juices, sprouts, raw nuts and seeds, 100% whole grain breads, pastas, cereals, beans and legumes. These are no-cholesterol, no-fat, no-salt, "live foods" that produce body fuel and help produce healthy, lively people. "Live foods" and fasting are the main reasons people become revitalized into a fresh new life filled with youthfulness, health, vitality, joy and longevity! There are millions of healthy Bragg followers worldwide proving this healthy lifestyle works!

The secret of longevity is eating and living intelligently. – Gayelord Hauser

Fasting breaks the addiction to junk food! Faithful fasting for only a few days can help break the addictions to tobacco, alcohol, drugs, coffee, soft drinks, and fast foods.

Vegetarianism Versus Meat Eating

Over the years that we've been Nutritionists, the controversy of "Vegetarianism vs. Meat Eating" has raged furiously. Both sides present the scientific reasons for their side. And we are not going to try to persuade you to be either a vegetarian or a meat eater. That is your choice. There are hundreds of books written on both subjects. Today scientific research has strongly established that a healthy vegetarian diet can play a major role in achieving optimal health and longevity! There are great health benefits for those who choose to follow a vegetarian life. Healthy vegetarian diets are optimal in heart disease prevention. Vegetarians have reduced cancer rates. Studies show vegetarians have increased longevity compared to meat eaters. Also check out these websites: *pcrm.org; vrg.org; VeganOutreach.org*

Bragg Prefers Healthier Vegetarian Diet

Over the years of following a program of fasting and eating a diet containing an abundance of raw organic fruits and vegetables, our bodies have become so keen that they practically tell us what to eat at every meal. After years on this healthy vegetarian diet, our bodies have lost the desire for meat, fowl and fish. Our diet is composed of raw organic fruits, vegetables, salads, sprouts, cooked vegetables, beans, legumes, brown rice, raw nuts and seeds and their butters, and nutritional yeast flakes. This is what our miracle bodies like to thrive on. Occasionally there were times when our bodies told us to eat a piece of meat or fish, or to have natural cheese or a few fertile eggs. In other words, our bodies developed an instinct for healthy foods. Sometimes we would go years without tasting eggs, and then our bodies would tell us that we need some. Listening to our bodies inner voice helps us enormously.

Researchers have discovered the more healthy habits an individual practices, the longer they live and the healthier and fitter they are!
– Elizabeth Vierck, "Health Smart: Personal Plan to Living Longer"

Eat to live, not live to eat. Many dishes, many diseases.
– Benjamin Franklin

If you eat meat, it should be organically fed and not eaten more than 1 to 2 times per week. Fresh fish can be the least toxic of flesh proteins, but beware of fish from polluted waters! Eat wild caught fish, such as salmon and sardines. If you are unsure of the water the fish comes from, don't risk eating it. Avoid shellfish, such as shrimp, lobster and crayfish, because they are garbage-eating bottom-feeders. They eat decaying scum and refuse off the bottoms of sick oceans, lakes and rivers. Chickens and turkeys that are commercially mass fed are heavily drugged with antibiotics and hormones. Stick to organically grown only. Be selective, cautious and wise in your eating; seek the healthiest optimal food choices!

It's best that people do not eat pork or pork products. The pig is the only animal besides man that develops arteriosclerosis. This animal is so loaded with cholesterol that in cold weather, unprotected pigs become stiff, as though frozen solid. Pigs are often infected with a dangerous parasite which causes the disease trichinosis.

Our Beloved Health Teachers and Mentors

One of the greatest teachers and physicians in the science of body purification and nutrition was **Dr. John Tilden, M.D.**, of Denver. This great scientist will surely go down in history as one of the finest physicians. His programs included fasting and an abundance of fresh fruits and vegetables. He lived into his 90s and was active to the end of his long life keeping his patients healthy.

Another one of the finest doctors we have ever known, who specialized in nutrition, was the famed **Dr. John Harvey Kellogg, M.D.** He was the director for 60 years of the famous Battle Creek Health Sanitarium in Battle Creek, Michigan. Dr. Kellogg's Sanitarium specialized in a vegetarian diet and people from all around the world were restored to radiant health by following his health program. Paul Bragg had the privilege of studying under Dr. Kellogg, and deemed it one of the outstanding experiences of his early health career.

We also associated with **Dr. Bernarr Macfadden**, Father and Founder of the Physical Culture Movement Bernarr Macfadden tried vegetarianism for a time, but gradually went back to a mixed diet which included some meat and fish. He lived healthy and active to nearly 88 years of age and he believed in mixing proteins.

Over our many years in the health field, we have met many famous men and women who restored thousands of people to health through natural methods. In the 1920s Paul Bragg worked with **Dr. St. Louis Estes**, D.D.S., who was a pioneer and strict believer in the raw food diet. He saw many broken, weak, sick people restored to health by changing to a raw food diet.

Dr. Benedict Lust, M.D., N.D., was the Father and Founder of Naturopathy in America, and established in New York a great school of Naturopathy which educated and graduated thousands of Naturopathic doctors who have used and spread his health teachings around the world.

Dr. Henry Lindlahr, M.D., was a famous drugless physician who lobbied for the return to natural methods in the modern treatment and prevention of disease.

Professor Arnold Ehret was one of world's greatest food scientists. He was the discoverer and creator of "The Mucusless Diet Healing System," which is a strictly vegetarian regime. Paul Bragg knew many of Professor Ehret's students in their 80s and 90s, who were still enjoying vigorous, robust health by following his wise vegetarian health program.

The greatest force in the human body is the natural drive of the body to heal itself – but that force is not independent of the belief system. Everything begins with belief. What we believe is the most powerful option of all. – Norman Cousins, author, "Anatomy of an Illness"

A Harvard Study shows the strong importance of mind/body connections in your health. Improving your mind with meditation, prayer, relaxation, walking, yoga, healthy diet, some fasting and positive thinking brought amazing improvements.

Hippocrates relied upon diet, fasting and exercise rather than drugs.

Chapter 9

Fasting Fights and Removes Mucus

In our opinion most of man's problems stem from a clogging of the entire pipe system of the human body. Most of this clogging takes the form of a thick mucus.

How free are you of this mucus at this moment? Do you have a postnasal drip? Is there a slow dripping of mucus from your sinus cavities into the back of your mouth and down your throat? What about your nose? How much mucus are you carrying in your nasal passages? How many times a day do you use a tissue? How many times a day do you clear your throat? How often do you cough or spit up mucus and phlegm?

Every person living on the Standard American Diet has, more or less, a sticky mucus-clogged pipe system. This stored-up toxic mucus results from undigested, uneliminated, unnatural food substances and toxins that start accumulating from birth. This mucus not only clogs the nose, throat and lungs, but is also found in the 30-foot gastrointestinal tract that starts at the mouth and ends at the anus. Some suffer great distress (such as asthma) from heavy mucus in their sinus cavities. Get the mucus out – cough, spit or blow. Never recycle mucus! When it drops into your throat, mouth or lungs, cough and spit it out!!! Never swallow it!!! Your body workers have collected it – now you help and get it out! But the most mucus is often lodged in the lungs.

Pneumonia is one of the most deadly diseases. Mucus fills the lungs so you can't get enough air to purify the 5 to 8 quarts of blood which flows to the lungs for purification. Pneumonia kills more older people; they literally drown from mucus in their lungs.

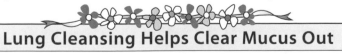

Lung Cleansing Helps Clear Mucus Out

Try this Lung Cleansing: Place 2-3 drops of "Oil of Oregano" (herbal oil) in 2 quarts of boiling water. Put a towel over your head and breathe in the vapors through the mouth and then your nose. This opens up the lungs. Do as needed 1-3 times daily.

The Standard American Diet Forms Mucus and Illness

The Standard American Diet (S.A.D.) is a mucus-forming, heavily refined, high sugar, salt, fried foods, meats, fats and dairy diet. Our bodies are equipped with an elastic pipe system. The modern diet that we eat is never entirely digested and the accumulated waste is never entirely eliminated. Our entire pipe system is slowly becoming clogged, especially the intestines and the digestive tract. This is the foundation of many physical problems. The body becomes overloaded with mucus which the avenues of elimination cannot expel. It concentrates into decayed, toxic masses. We call this the "Mucoid Plaque" on our intestines.

All dairy products are especially mucus-forming. No animal in the world except man drinks milk after being weaned. The modern diet includes butter, margarines, processed shortenings and hydrogenated fats and oils that are plugging saturated fats! These are unhealthy for the body. Our bodies have a normal body temperature of 98.6°F. To digest and assimilate these solid, hardened, saturated fats, we would have to heat our bodies to 300°F. The Standard American Diet contains loads of processed and synthetic cheese, as well as natural cheese which is heavily preserved with salt. Non-mineralized modern salt is dangerous to the body. Don't use it! Use sea salt or fully mineralized salt.

Mucus Shows Up in Urine When Fasting

The urine test shows the amount of mucus the average human carries within their bloodstream. When you are fasting, each morning of your fast take a sample of the first urine you pass on awakening, put in a labeled bottle, and place the bottle on a shelf to cool and settle. In a few days this urine will show a toxic cloud of mucus. The longer you store the urine, the more toxins will be revealed. A weekly 24-hour fast will help rid your body of large amounts of mucus and toxins. Some of these toxins have been circulating in your body for years.

In the winter, most people eat more heavy, concentrated foods – such as refined flour, pancakes, waffles, sugary doughnuts, rolls, breads, flour gravies, pies and refined pastas. The body then becomes so loaded with mucus that it forces the Vital Force to create a cleansing crisis – a cold or flu. A fever is produced by your Vital Force to help burn up and flush out heavy concentrations of mucus. The lungs, nose and throat pour out mucus through coughing, sneezing, spitting and nose-blowing. Few humans realize what a cleansing the body goes through!

The body is a miracle self-purifying instrument! As long as the body has enough Vital Force to eliminate toxins such as mucus, it will work with all its energy to rid and purify the body! What do humans think about this crisis? They get feverish. A fever is your body's cleaner, a natural phenomenon of Mother Nature that is acting as an incinerator to burn up all the toxins!

Do A Mucus Test – It Will Amaze You!

You can start a mucus test by eliminating all of the mucus-forming foods from your diet for several months. Fast 1 day a week and, if possible, build up to a 3-4 or 7-day fast. Watch your urine closely. See for yourself the amount of mucus you have concentrated in your body. After a fast, make 60% to 70% of your diet raw salads, vegetables and fruits and the balance in cooked vegetables, beans, legumes and brown rice. This is a mucusless diet that's rich in enzymes and nutrients. Also the raw, unsalted nuts and nut butters and seeds (almond, pumpkin, sunflower, walnuts) are not mucus-forming, so you can add them to your diet of organic fruits and vegetables. While on this test do not eat any dairy, eggs, meats and only a few whole grains or none at all.

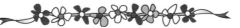

HEALTHY MIND HABITS: Wake up and say – "Today I am going to be happier, healthier and wiser in my daily living! I am the captain of my life and I am going to steer it living a 100% healthy lifestyle!" Happy people look younger, are healthier and live longer!
– Patricia Bragg

We can tell you all the great health benefits that fasting, and a mucusless and meatless diet will do for you! But it's best that you simply try it for yourself and be the judge! Notice how seldom you have mucus and have to use a tissue. A 7-day fast is a great mucus eliminator. We make it a practice to fast 7 to 10 days in late October or November so that, as the winter comes on, we have relieved our body of any mucus that has accumulated. We try to live on a mucusless diet! When traveling the world lecturing, we had found at times we couldn't get all the organic fruits and vegetables we normally eat, so we put our faith in fasting for needed purification.

After the first 2 or 3 days of fasting you will notice that you are no longer hungry. From the third day on there is no craving for food. When people go on crash low calorie diets, they are hungry most of the time and long for heavy meals. But after you fast for 2 or 3 days, hunger fades away, the stomach shrinks and it becomes a pleasant experience! You start to breathe easier, feel lighter, move easier, think clearer and then miracles start happening!

Fasting Rewards You With Increased Energy

We have seen many people lose 7 to 20 pounds and more the first 7 to 10 days of fasting. After the loss of this excess weight, there is a special inner feeling of well-being and increased physical and mental energy! Of course, every human is different. Some people will only lose 1 or 2 pounds a day on a fast while others will lose as many as 5 pounds and more. The nice thing about fasting to reduce is that the pounds will disappear where the fat is deposited. If the weight has concentrated on the abdomen and hips, that is where the fat will shrink. Many times the people who go on a low calorie diet end up feeling miserable while they are dieting. They become haggard and old-looking and their eyes will lose their sparkle. It's just the reverse when you fast. **The fat deposits dissolve first and – as the body is relieved of this tremendous burden of toxins – the heart, pulse, blood pressure and general health regulate themselves.**

You can transition to a weekly 24-hour fasting program gently and easily. We often supervise weight reduction programs, where we direct people on several 36-hour fasts in a week. In other words, the person will eat one day, and then fast a day or fast every third day. If the person doesn't overload themselves on the days that they eat, the 36-hour fast several days a week or every fourth day helps maintain the weight loss. **Fasting for weight reduction gets results! Your body will soon slim and trim itself back to its healthy, youthful fit self.**

Your Waistline is Your Lifeline & Dateline!

We have had years of experience in fasting many of our greatest film and television Stars in Hollywood. The movie camera always makes a person look 10 pounds heavier than they really are, so you can see that a Hollywood Star must always try to have slim, trim lines!

We recall a well-known female movie star who struggled with compulsive eating because she was having marital and financial troubles. She sought solace in rich foods such as ice cream, sugared pastries and candies. She lost her movie contract. She lost her confidence. This actress became depressed and she was sent to us for guidance. We explained to her that it had taken months for her to add this weight to her body and it would now take time to slim, trim and normalize her weight! **She was determined so she was cooperative!**

First, we put her on a healthy, balanced diet program with fruit for breakfast, and for lunch a raw salad with 2 lightly cooked vegetables. We took all breads, cereals and animal proteins out of her diet. In the evening she had the *Raw Health Salad* and *Brown Rice & Lentil Casserole* (recipe page 125). We had her eliminate all refined white sugar desserts!

Fasting and hunger helps energize and activate the body and mind. With Fasting there is no detrimental effect on cognitive performance, activity, sleep or mood. – Jason Fung, M.D., "The Complete Guide to Fasting"

 True wisdom is to know what is best worth knowing, and to do what is best worth doing. – Edward Humphrey

We started her on 2 weekly 24-hour fasts for the first 2 weeks. The third week we gave her a 3-day fast and the fifth week we gave her a full 7-day fast. After a month of healthy eating we put her on a 10-day fast. We had her eat for 2 weeks and then we put her on a 15-day fast. This eating, then fasting program did the trick! She got back her lovely figure. Her eyes became bright and clear and she regained her youthful, sparkling appearance. Most of all her self-esteem and self-respect and self-confidence. Producers and directors, and her many friends were amazed.

Fasting is the Healthiest, Fastest Weight Normalizer

Fasting works miracles for both the under and overweight! The genuine needs for both types of people are met by exactly the same program of natural living combined with fasting.

Fasting is the magic key for helping anyone to restore themselves to a natural state of health. Fasting is the great detoxifier and by detoxifying the body we give it a chance to restore its natural functioning. **Fasting is the great "Open Sesame" to good health and a long life.**

Each person is different and some people get results quicker than others! If you faithfully concentrate on living *The Bragg Healthy Lifestyle* in which fasting plays an integral part, Mother Nature will not fail you! So, if you are thin, underweight and have tried various weight-building diets that failed, don't be discouraged. Try a 24-hour fast weekly and the apple cider vinegar drink (see recipe page 124). Both will help give your precious body a chance to cleanse and normalize your weight.

The doctor of the future will give no medicine, but will interest her or his patients in the care of the human frame, in a proper diet and in the cause and prevention of disease. – Thomas Edison

We love helping people who want to live and follow *The Bragg Healthy Lifestyle*! We want to help you now!

Chapter 10

Fasting Fights Winter Miseries

No matter how well and healthy you try to live, colds, sniffles and flus will catch up with you. If this happens, please don't be discouraged, but be thankful your body is house cleaning and pushing out debris and toxins.

When your nose drips watery mucus and your head feels thick while you sneeze; when fever burns through your body and you feel terrible, don't blame it on the weather or on a cold draft of air! Don't blame it on the fact that your feet got wet or chilled! And above all, please don't say, *"I caught this!"* The proper name for this is, *"I have an acute healing crisis."* The reason we go through this is that we live in a complex civilization and we have lost so much of our natural health instinct to keep internally pure. Our environment is so much more toxic, than was the environment of our grandparents, great-grandparents and our ancestors.

51

For some physiological reason that is unexplainable the Vital Force within our bodies loosens up waste, toxins and mucus and proceeds to get rid of it with what we call an *"acute healing crisis"* also known as a cold or a flu. If you cooperate with your Vital Force, this rough spot in your life will pass quickly. Just understand that your Vital Force is trying to keep you internally clean!

If you interfere with wise Mother Nature, you'll complicate the natural procedure of your body's miraculous cleansing job. Now that you know why this is occurring, do nothing to stop this cleansing process except to fast. Fresh vegetable juices, warm broths, herbal teas. Yes, that's the best answer. Fast and help your body cleanse and be healthy.

You must not fight this healing crisis because Mother Nature knows what she is doing for you. What should you do? Start your fasting program right away! There is absolutely nothing as important as your health and life!

Fasting is a Miraculous Rebirth and Resurrection!

Let us tell you naturally what fasting can do for you. This natural miracle will help reverse the premature ageing process. From this minute on, you will take a new lease on life! It has been proven by some of the world's greatest scientists that fasting is the magic key that opens the door to agelessness and youthfulness.

Scientists have been experimenting for years on worms, rats, and guinea pigs, and discovered remarkable scientific facts. They fasted these lab specimens and, in between fast periods, fed them natural diets. A miracle occurred, they got younger, some tripled their life span! These scientists wanted only facts that revealed the truth! Fasting slows down the ageing clock, and produces a healthy youthfulness and rebirth in the body. In all the fasts we have supervised, we have seen millions of unbelievable miracles happen to people of all ages.

52 Recharged, So at 70 A World Tennis Champ

Martin Cornica learned the same facts that we have shared with millions around the world. When you know the science of taking care of the body, you have the secret of a naturally healthy and youthful life. Martin longed to look and feel youthful! He was eager to try Mother Nature's plan of living as we taught him.

He went on a 24-hour fast the day after he attended The Bragg Health Crusade. He began to eat a healthy and perfectly balanced diet. **Through fasting and The Bragg Healthy Lifestyle he dropped years from his age!** Even though he was 40 years old and considered long past the age to play champion tennis, Mr. Cornica felt stronger than when he was 20! His energy and vitality was super, so he joined the famous Los Angeles Tennis Club and started to play tennis again.

My dear friend, I know your soul is doing fine and I pray that you are doing well in every way and that your health is good. – 3 John 2

He continued his weekly 24-hour fast and lived on a natural food diet. Every day he improved in every way! His endurance soon was so great that he was playing the champion tennis players of the world! For the next 30 years he played in one major tournament after another and won many championships! Tennis is often seen as a game for only the young, but here was a man supposedly long past his prime playing young champions and winning!

Martin Cornica became The Champion Tennis Player of the World for all men over 70! People in the tennis world were completely amazed when they saw this man in his 70s playing a smashing championship game of tennis.

The average person believes that by the time a man is 70 he is either half dead or used up. Martin Cornica is living proof that this is a fallacy! It's not the number of years you live on this earth, it's how you live your years! We are so proud because he has proven that anyone can attain agelessness and be reborn by following Mother Nature's Laws of Living. Regardless of your age, Mother Nature will give you the opportunity to make a comeback. Yes, you can step out of that tired, prematurely ageing body and rebuild a strong body that will become healthier and more youthful everyday!

After a year of periodic fasting combined with living *The Bragg Healthy Lifestyle*, you will look in the mirror and be happy with the great improvement you have made. If you continue to live *The Bragg Healthy Lifestyle* as described in this book, the physical transformation will make your friends and relatives take notice and marvel. You will not only see the difference in yourself, you will feel the difference! But only you can make this metamorphosis if you are willing to exercise absolute mastery of your entire body.

Everyday is a birthday; every moment of it is new to us; we are born again; renewed for fresh work and endeavor. – Isaac Watts

---

 Fasting is for internal cleansing, purification to stay healthy and youthful.

Start as Martin Cornica did with a 24-hour fast. The *Nine Doctors of Mother Nature* that we speak of in the chapters ahead will aid you in your rebirth! They are always ready and willing to help those who help themselves. As you get younger and more vital, you may see those you love begin to decay and pass out of your life. The same thing has happened to us. We have had to watch many friends that we loved get sick, suffer and die long before their time because they did not live a healthy lifestyle. *Smoking got our friends – our dear friends – Walt Disney, John Wayne, Clark Gable and Lana Turner.*

We challenge you. Here's the opportunity of your lifetime. Revolt! Refuse to grow old and lose any of your precious years. Mother Nature is waiting for you to make your positive decision NOW!

You have decided to take the *Bragg Health and Happiness Road* to super health! There might be a few rough spots as you begin, but soon you will be hiking along the highway of health and long-lasting youthfulness!

54

You can't fail when you are working with Mother Nature – a force that wants you to be healthy and fulfilled. Begin your 24-hour fast today, and soon you will be laughing at birthdays. They will mean nothing to you! Because you are living in the blessed state of agelessness.

The Bragg Health & Happiness Plan

- *Read, plan, plot, and follow through for supreme health and longevity.*
- *Underline, highlight or dog-ear pages as you read important passages.*
- *Organizing your lifestyle helps you identify what's important in your life.*
- *Be faithful to your health goals everyday for a healthy, long, happy life.*
- *Where space allows we include "words of wisdom" from great minds to motivate and inspire you. Please share your favorite sayings with us.*
- *Do write us about your successes following The Miracle of Fasting.*

Please copy and cut out – for you to fold and keep in your wallet.

Patricia's "Angel Gift" to You

Here's your own "Pocket Angel" to be with you night and day – to guide, protect, and show you right from wrong, and help you heal your life . . . physically, mentally, emotionally and spiritually with Angel Love.

Chapter 11

Fasting Keeps
Arteries Youthful

Cardiovascular disease is responsible for 25% of the deaths in the United States, according to the American Heart Association. This alarms all of us! Often we are shocked to hear that 224 people have died in an airplane crash, but we are blasé about the fact that every day over 4,000 Americans die from heart disease! **Disease of the heart, arteries and blood vessels is not only an epidemic in America, it's the #1 killer! This enemy of mankind targets men and women, old and young! More than 1 in 4 Americans are currently suffering from some form of cardiovascular disease!** Even during the Korean, Vietnam, Gulf Wars, and current wars, autopsies revealed that many young service people suffered from deteriorated and degenerated arteries – sadly, long before their time!

Diseases of the heart do not build up rapidly. It takes a long time to harden and block an artery! Heart disease has many causes: tobacco, alcohol, unhealthy diet – heavy in hydrogenated and saturated trans fats as in fast foods, meats, dairy products – and the lack of exercise! **Heart disease is often a silent killer! Too frequently, blockage in the arteries builds up to the danger point while the victim is totally unaware!** It's possible for a person to have half-blocked arteries all over their body without the slightest indication that anything is wrong! This person might even receive a clean bill of health from the best doctors! This happened to American President Dwight D. Eisenhower – 1 week after a thorough physical with a good health report, he had a major heart attack and almost died!

55

Shocking Heart Facts About The #1 Killer

- 1.5 million Americans will have a new or recurrent heart attack and about 610,000 of them will die each year – that's 1 in every 4 deaths!
- Every 40 seconds another American dies from cardiovascular disease!
- Heart disease doesn't just kill the old; 45% occurs in people under 65!
- Heart disease affects both men and women; 27% of men and 44% of women will die within 1 year after having a heart attack.

The substances responsible for obstructing the arteries are cholesterol, fats, inorganic minerals and fibrous tissues. As the blockage builds up slowly, the inner passages of the arteries can become so narrow that not enough blood can flow through to properly nourish that powerful heart muscle! Coronary occlusion is caused when this serious narrowing of the arteries occurs!

You Are as Old as Your Arteries!

Degeneration of the arteries begins early in life, slowly building up to obstruct and block! And then, one fine morning, someone gets up as usual to start the day's activities and, in the blink of an eye, they drop dead from a heart attack or if they survive, they live with a very serious health condition.

Constant health vigilance must be maintained if the arteries are to be kept free of blockage and obstruction by substances that can cause a heart attack. The heart arteries are small; the largest is no wider than a thin soda straw. In the average person who eats the Standard American Diet, the blockage grows silently, insidiously until the blood can no longer flow freely through the arteries and then disaster strikes in a heart attack or a stroke.

Most people wait until something happens to their arteries before they do anything about it. Because no pains are evident, they continue to eat bad foods and live with unhealthy habits!

Let us repeat the statement, *"We are all as old as our arteries."* Remember that arterial blockage starts even in the very young and slowly builds up until around 50 to 70 years of age, when most heart attacks happen.

We want it definitely understood that fasting is not a cure for heart problems. Fasting is a cleanser of internal impurities! This is exactly how we want to help the arteries – to keep them clean and free of substances that prevent the free flow of blood into the heart and throughout the entire arterial system.

Don't let cardiovascular disease affect you! Protect your heart!
Faithfully live The Bragg Healthy Lifestyle – please start now!

Body's Main Nourishing Arteries & Veins –
A Walking, Talking, Human Miracle Machine

Arteries

Veins

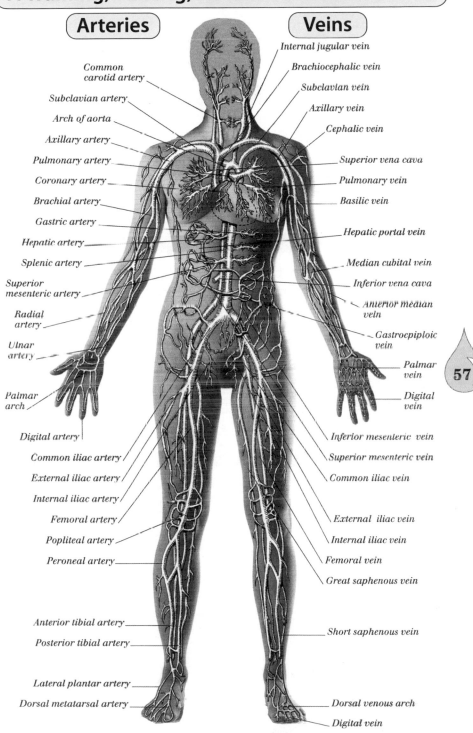

Common carotid artery

Subclavian artery

Arch of aorta

Axillary artery

Pulmonary artery

Coronary artery

Brachial artery

Gastric artery

Hepatic artery

Splenic artery

Superior mesenteric artery

Radial artery

Ulnar artery

Palmar arch

Digital artery

Common iliac artery

External iliac artery

Internal iliac artery

Femoral artery

Popliteal artery

Peroneal artery

Anterior tibial artery

Posterior tibial artery

Lateral plantar artery

Dorsal metatarsal artery

Internal jugular vein

Brachiocephalic vein

Subclavian vein

Axillary vein

Cephalic vein

Superior vena cava

Pulmonary vein

Basilic vein

Hepatic portal vein

Median cubital vein

Inferior vena cava

Anterior median vein

Gastroepiploic vein

Palmar vein

Digital vein

Inferior mesenteric vein

Superior mesenteric vein

Common iliac vein

External iliac vein

Internal iliac vein

Femoral vein

Great saphenous vein

Short saphenous vein

Dorsal venous arch

Digital vein

57

Remember Your Precious Body is A Miracle!
– *Patricia Bragg, Pioneer Health Crusader*

What You Eat and Drink Becomes You

We have, in the final analysis, a human pipe system that carries our precious five quarts of blood throughout the entire circulatory system. Our blood circulation must be kept constantly moving, rhythmically and steadily. For instance, if the flow of blood into the brain is stopped for a fraction of a minute, we would suffer a massive stroke. If it happens in the eye, hemorrhaging can occur that may blind us. The arteries must remain open so the bloodstream will flow to every square inch of the body!

Today you will find men and women in their 70s, 80s and even 90s who have clear, clean, unobstructed, elastic and flexible arteries. Regardless of their calendar years, they are young and active because their arteries have not degenerated to the point of becoming obstructed and inflexible. These are the most fortunate people in the world because if all the organs of their bodies are free from obstruction and toxic materials, there is no reason why these ageless people cannot live a long life!

Your Miracle Heart and Circulatory System

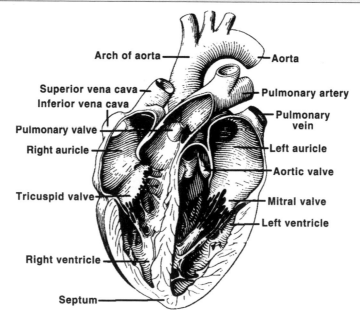

Arch of aorta — — Aorta
Superior vena cava — — Pulmonary artery
Inferior vena cava
— Pulmonary vein
Pulmonary valve — — Left auricle
Right auricle — — Aortic valve
Tricuspid valve — — Mitral valve
— Left ventricle
Right ventricle —
Septum —

The heart is really a double pump – each side is composed of two powerful chambers, an auricle and a ventricle.

Eat Healthy – Live Healthy – Live Longer

When we fast from a 24-to 36-hour period, or from 3 to 10 days, all the Vital Force in the body is used for internal purification and cleansing, especially the arteries. That is why after a 10-day fast there's a feeling of lightness in the body! The mind becomes keener, more loving, alert and all memory improves. The craving for physical activity will become intense. Fasting helps to keep the arteries clean, elastic and more youthful.

We reiterate the importance of a thorough check of the urine. During the 10-day fast, daily the first morning urine can be bottled, labeled and saved for observation. The faster will note the amount of foreign substances that are being eliminated from the body, particularly the mucus toxins that appear in the urine.

In our opinion, we can add years to our hearts with a systematic program of fasting, coupled with *The Bragg Healthy Lifestyle Program* of natural food which reduces the waxy cholesterol that clogs arteries. We must think of our arteries as the key to life if we want to win the greatest battle in life – which is staying alive on this earth! When we eat high-fat, fast food meals day after day we are bound to accumulate cholesterol, obstructions and toxins. Americans are the world's biggest eaters of fat! Consequently we lead the world in cardiovascular, heart and stroke diseases.

This is one reason that we believe in the *"No Heavy Breakfast Plan"* (see page 19) also known as intermittent fasting. We have known many healthy, young men and women who made it a habit every morning of eating a so-called hearty breakfast of ham and eggs or bacon and eggs, buttered toast, fried potatoes and coffee loaded with cream. Many of these supposedly healthy people were stricken with early heart attacks or strokes that either killed them or made them invalids for the rest of their lives. We always say, *"You are what you eat, drink, breathe, think, say and do!"*

Dr. Dean Ornish can reverse heart disease in over 70% of his patients who follow, among other things, a low-fat vegetarian diet. Dr. Ornish's program optimizes four important areas of your life. His program deals with the root causes not just its effects. – See web: DeanOrnish.com

HEALTHY HEART HABITS FOR LONG, VITAL LIFE

Remember, *organic live foods make live people. You are what you eat, drink, breathe, think, say and do.* So eat a low-fat, low-sugar, high-fiber diet of organic fresh raw salads, sprouts, greens, vegetables, whole grains, fruits, raw seeds, nuts, fresh juices and chemical-free, purified or distilled water.

Earn your food with daily exercise. For regular exercise, brisk walking, improves your health, stamina, go-power, flexibility, endurance and helps open the cardiovascular system! Only 45 minutes a day truly can do miracles for your heart, arteries, mind, nerves, soul and body! You become revitalized with new zest for living to accomplish your life goals!

We are made of tubes. To help keep them open, clean and to maintain good elimination, I take 1 veg psyllium cap or add 1 tsp psyllium husk powder daily an hour after dinner to juices, herbal teas, even apple cider vinegar drink. I also take one Cayenne capsule (40,000 HU) daily with a meal. I also take 50 to 100 mgs. regular-released Niacin (B3) with one meal daily to help cleanse and open the cardiovascular system; also improves memory. Skin flushing may occur, don't worry about this as it shows it's working! After cholesterol level reaches 180, then only take Niacin twice weekly.

The heart needs healthy balanced nutrients, so take natural multi-vitamin-mineral food supplements: Omega-3 and extra heart helpers – vitamin E with mixed tocotrienols; vitamin C; Ubiquinol CoQ10; vitamin D3; MSM; D-Ribose; garlic; turmeric; selenium; zinc; beta carotene and amino acids – L-Carnitine, L-Taurine, L-Lysine and Proline. Folic acid, CoQ10, vitamin B6 and B12 helps keep homocysteine level low. Magnesium orotate, hawthorn berry extract helps bring relief for palpitations, arrhythmia, senile hearts and coronary disease. Take multi-digestive enzyme and probiotics with meals; it aids in digestion, assimilation and elimination.

For sleep problems try 5-HTP tryptophan (an amino acid), melatonin, calcium, magnesium, valerian (in capsule, extract or tea), and Sleepytime herb tea. For arthritis or joint pain/stiffness, try aloe juice or gel, glucosamine-chondroitin-MSM combo caps and shots, helps heal and regenerate. Capsaicin and DMSO lotion helps relieve pain. Natural liver cleanses to repair and regenerate include: milk thistle; dandelion root; artichoke and turmeric. Dandelion root is a natural diuretic and helps clear toxins through urination and also helps stimulate liver bile flow so waste can be eliminated.

Use amazing antioxidants – E Tocotrienols, vitamin C, quercetin, grape seed extract (OPCs), CoQ10, selenium, SOD, resveratrol, and alpha-lipoic acid. They improve immune system and help flush out dangerous free radicals that cause havoc with cardiovascular pipes and health. Research shows antioxidants promote longevity, slow ageing, fight toxins, help prevent disease, cancer, cataracts and exhaustion.

Recommended Heart Health Tests (for Adults):

- **Total Cholesterol:** 180 mg/dl or less is optimal
- **LDL Cholesterol:** 130 mg/dl or less is optimal • **HDL Cholesterol:** 50 mg/dl or more
- **Triglycerides:** 150 mg/dl or less is normal level
- **HDL/Cholesterol Ratio:** 5.0 or less • **Triglycerides/HDL Ratio:** below 2
- **Homocysteine:** 6-9 micromoles/L
- **CRP (C-Reactive Protein high sensitivity):**
  - 1 mg/L = low risk • 1-3 mg/L = average risk • over 3 mg/L = high risk
- **Diabetic Risk Tests:**
  - **Glucose:** (do 12 hour food fast) 80-100 mg/dl • **Hemoglobin A1c:** 6% or less
- **Blood Pressure:** 120/70 mmHg is good for adults

Chapter 12

Nine Health Doctors At Your Command

- Sunshine • Fresh Air • Pure Water
- Healthy Natural Foods • Fasting • Exercise
- Rest • Good Posture • Strong Human Mind

Mother Nature's nine faithful *"Health Doctors"* are ready to help you attain radiant, glorious health! They're all specialists in their particular fields of health building. They have had centuries of proven experience with millions. Their cumulative record is 100% perfect! They have never failed a patient. But we have failed them. We have turned our backs on them and ignored them! But they are kind, patient and understanding, no matter how many times we have failed them, they stand ready to render perfect professional service. And they have but one prescription and that is the elixir of life! They are the gentlest doctors in the whole universe! They are anxious and willing to help everyone who comes to them for Higher Health. Their professional services are available to all of us – the young, the old, the rich and the poor. They perform no operations, except bloodless ones. They give no toxic, harmful drugs, not even any so-called "wonder drugs."

61

We are all familiar with these nine wonderful life-changing "Health Doctors" – and we all need them! We want you to call on them frequently! They are eager to help you help yourself!

These wonderful "Doctors" do not want you to be sick! They want you to be healthy and they want to be your personal care-givers and friends. It gives us a most secure feeling that we have at our command every day, the world's great "Doctors" and it is our pleasure to introduce you to them. From this day on, please feel free to call on them. First, we want you to meet the Father of them all, the most eminent and greatest healer and giver of life to everything on the face of this earth . . . **Doctor Sunshine.**

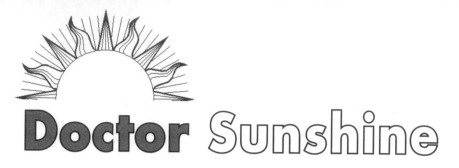

Doctor Sunshine

Doctor Sunshine's specialty is heliotherapy and his great prescription is solar energy! Each tiny blade of grass, every vine, tree, bush, flower, fruit and vegetable draws its life from solar energy. All living things on earth depend on solar energy, the source of all life. This earth would be a barren, frigid place if it were not for sunshine. There would be no you and no me. Sadly the earth would be in everlasting darkness.

Human beings were never meant to have pale skins, not even the fairest northern races. Man's skin should be tanned slightly by the sun and take on a darker pigment than his original skin tone. It has been found that even fair, red-headed people can slowly tan. Pigmentation is a sign that solar energy has been transformed into human energy. By safely enjoying the early morning or late afternoon gentle sunshine we can gain more health, vitality and happiness.

The person who is starved of the vital rays of the sun has a half-dead look, and is actually dying for the want of solar energy! Weak, ailing and anemic people are sun-starved and – in our opinion – **many people are sick simply because they are starving for gentle sunshine.**

The sunshine's gentlest rays have powerful germicidal properties. As the skin gathers these gentle rays, it stores up enormous amounts of a germ-killing energy. The sun provides one of the finest remedies for the nervous person who is filled with anxiety, worry and frustration.

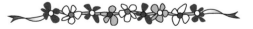

 Doctor Sunshine gives us Vitamin D – the great healer, soothes and sparkles your body inside and outside!
– Paul C. Bragg, N.D., Ph.D., Pioneer Life Extension Specialist

Chapter 13

Doctor Fresh Air

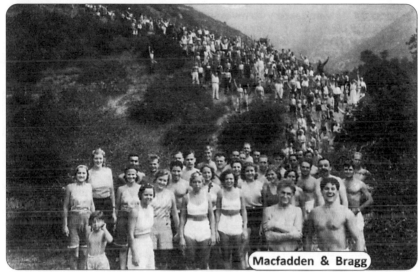

Macfadden & Bragg

Bragg Health Students enjoying hiking, exercise and the fresh air on a trail to Mt. Hollywood, California, summer of 1932.

Doctor Fresh Air is a health specialist, and his greatest prescription for you is to "Breathe Deeply of Mother Nature's Fresh Air." The first thing we do when we are born is take a long, deep breath and the last thing we do is take a last gasp before we stop breathing. Between birth and death, life is completely maintained by breathing. Doctor Fresh Air wants you to have a long active life and as a specialist, feels that if you will follow his simple instructions and breathe deeply, you will have a healthy long life! You must always be conscious that with every breath you take, you are bringing into your body the Breath of Mother Nature . . . life-giving oxygen! When we fail to obey this doctor's orders about getting plenty of fresh air every day and night we are inviting some severe complications.

Breathing deeply, fully and completely energizes the body, calms the nerves, fills you with peace and helps keep you youthful. – Paul C. Bragg

Our Body is a Breathing Miracle Machine

Let us examine closely the function of breathing. **Every living thing breathes in oxygen, the body's miracle invisible food! It's the only food we cannot be deprived of for over 7 minutes or death will take us.** We not only receive life-giving oxygen that is necessary to every cell in our bodies from the air, but when we breathe, oxygen is carried by the blood to the lungs where a miracle takes place. There life-giving oxygen is exchanged for deadly carbon dioxide, in which form many of the deadly toxins of the body are released. In other words, we create toxic poisons in our body during the process of living. These are collected by the blood as it circulates and, after the blood brings carbon dioxide to the lungs, it's expelled as the new life-giving oxygen enters. Carbon dioxide is also burned up through the process of metabolism and during the creation and destruction of the cells of the body.

When we don't get enough fresh air – or if we are a shallow breather – and the oxygen intake doesn't equal the outgo of carbon dioxide, then these toxic poisons can build up within the body structure. This can result in serious physical problems as the retained carbon dioxide can concentrate in other parts of the body to cause intense physical suffering.

Enervation, which is the lack of nerve energy, can lower the Vital Force so much that the body's great bellows – the lungs – cannot pump in enough air to flush carbon dioxide out of the body. We can see how important it is that we not only breathe fresh, clean air, but we are conscious that we breathe deeply in and out!

We are miracle air machines! Oxygen not only purifies the body, but it is one of the great energizers. Our bodies are air pressure machines. We live at the bottom of an atmospheric ocean approximately 70 miles deep. The air pressure is 14 pounds per square inch. Between the inhalation and the exhalation of a breath, a vacuum is formed. As long as we continue to have this rhythmical intake and output of oxygen, we will live. We can go without food for 30 days or more and still survive, but we can only go without air for a few minutes.

The Importance of Clean Air to Health

It's essential to breathe clean air – air that's as free as possible from such chemicals as smog, car exhaust, natural gas appliance fumes and the many other toxic chemical pollutants. Also, our air needs to be as free as possible from mold, dust, dust mites and their fecal matter, animal dander and pollen! Everyone's health is helped in varying degrees by clean air. It's vitally important to live and work in an area which has clean air and is free of all harmful fumes. It's also equally important to keep our homes pure, clean and free from dust, dust mites and debris! Most people cannot be truly 100% healthy until they breathe clean air, maintain a healthy diet and live a healthy lifestyle.

Live Longer Breathing Clean Air Deeply

We advise those who have to live or work in smoggy, polluted cities to obtain a good air filter. We especially recommend filters which contain charcoal and a high efficiency particulate HEPA air filter. The charcoal removes most of the chemicals and the HEPA filter removes most of the particles. To be effective in an average room, the flow rate through the filter should be over 200 cubic feet of air per minute. A wise motorist will also install an air filter in his car.

When we are born, our lungs are new, fresh, clean, and rosy in color! If we could live in a pollutant and dust-free atmosphere breathing deeply all our lives, our lungs would remain *as good as new* for a long life of use. Yet many people abuse their lungs! Some of this comes from external causes. The lungs and skin are not the only organs of the body that are directly affected by external conditions, but the lungs are specifically effected by environmental toxins!

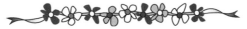

Life is in the breath. He who half breathes, half lives! – Old Proverb

Your breathing habits are the first place one should look when fatigue, disease or other evidence of disordered energy presents itself.
– Dr. Sheldon Hendler, "The Oxygen Breakthrough"

Deep Breathing Builds A Powerful Body

So, along with your fasting program, make it a point every day of your life to have a brisk two to five mile walk and, during that walk, breathe deeply. Every time you think of it during your waking hours, take long, slow, deep breaths. Remember what we have told you – the more long, slow, deep breaths you take, the longer and healthier you will live! When you combine deep breathing with fasting you are adding years to your life! You are building energy and vitality. Remind yourself daily that Doctor Fresh Air is your invisible staff of life and your constant friend.

Mechanics of Breathing

The mechanics of breathing, showing the position of the diaphragm and ribs at exhalation and at inhalation.

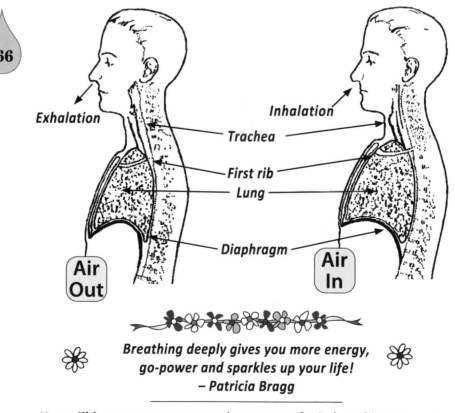

Exhalation

Inhalation

Trachea

First rib

Lung

Diaphragm

Air Out

Air In

Breathing deeply gives you more energy, go-power and sparkles up your life!
– Patricia Bragg

You will increase your energy, joy, peace of mind, and improve your health, (sleep too) with more daily exercise and deep breathing.

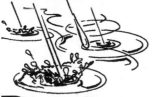

Doctor Pure Water

The Water You Drink
Can Make or Break Your Health!

Doctor Pure Water is a vitally important healer and splendid friend. Water is involved in nearly every physical process (see page 69). Water makes up about 75% of our body, so we need a continuous replacement to keep our water levels normal and healthy. Optimal is 8-10 large glasses of water daily. When we eat organic fruits and veggies we are also adding their liquids, distilled by nature, to our healthy diet.

There's so many health benefits from water that you can enjoy. A warm bath is a tonic and a relaxer which soothes irritated nerves and quiets our emotions. Every day of the year in the United States people enjoy swimming in water at the seashore, lakes, rivers, streams and swimming pools. Swimming is one of the best, most gentle exercises anyone can perform. It puts no strain on the joints or the heart. Swim as often as you can. If you don't know how to swim, go to a professional who can teach you. You will never regret it because it is one of the most relaxing and exhilarating exercises. It can be enjoyed at any age.

Water therapies have been used for man's miseries since the beginning of time. In our world travels we have found many different types of water therapies. It's been proven that the ancient civilizations of the Egyptians, Assyrians, Hebrews, Persians, Greeks, Hindus, Chinese and other cultures, including the Native American Indians, have used water therapies for the relief of human body ailments.

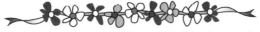

The power of pure water is the vital chemistry of your life!

The noblest of the elements is pure water. – Pindar, Greek Poet 443 B.C.

Chapter 14

Most Ancient Healers Used Water Therapy

In 400 B.C. – 400 years before the birth of Christ, on the Greek island of Kos in the Aegean Sea, Hippocrates, the father of medicine, developed a complete system of water treatments. His records state that a cold bath followed by a hot bath and a massage improves circulation. We agree! A cold and then a hot bath followed by a coarse friction rub is one of the best circulation healers. And other people enjoy a hot bath followed by a cold rush of water to awaken them for the day.

We do not regard hot mineral water as a cure for any human ailment. But we do believe that hot water, particularly at 104°F, is a purifier and a detoxifier that increases the body's circulation! That is why we recommend a hot Epsom salt bath or apple cider vinegar bath (1 cup) as a detoxifier and relaxer. It should be taken in bath water anywhere from 98°F to 104°F, for 10-15 minutes. This special bath can be a very important part of your health program. Usually it's best not to take an overly hot bath during your fasts, but warm water is okay.

Always remember that clean, pure water inside and out is the best to use. It's one of Mother Nature's wonderful ways of building a healthy body. Distilled water is the purest and the best for drinking and all food uses.

Water is More Important Than Food

More than 75% of the human body is water. The bones in your body are even 31% water. To lose a tenth of your body's water supply is dangerous, and to lose a fifth can be fatal. Losing lesser amounts disturbs bodily functions and impairs chemical and physical processes necessary to good health. Yet the body itself can take lots of punishment. Half your proteins and almost all of your fat and glycogen can be lost without causing death. Only that important 75% of your body level of water requires that it be kept at a consistently high level.

Pure water is the best drink for a wise man. – Henry David Thoreau

68

A practical example of the body's demand for water can be drawn from mountain climbing histories. In their assault on the Himalayas, men working and climbing in high altitudes cut down on the weight they carried in an attempt to conserve body energy. None were notably successful until a team conquering Mount Everest had scientifically considered the effect of the altitude on the body's water metabolism. These men increased their fuel load in order to melt snow and ice into water (distilled of course). They were assured of an average of 6 pints of water daily per person. While water was not the sole contributing factor to their success, it was recognized as helping to prevent fatigue experienced by former teams during their final assaults. The rest of us may not need water for anything as demanding as climbing the Himalayas, but this is an example of how important water – or the lack of it – in our diets can be.

WATER IS KEY TO HEALTH & ALL BODILY FUNCTIONS:

- Heart
- Circulation
- Digestion
- Bones & Joints
- Muscles
- Metabolism
- Assimilation
- Elimination
- Nerves
- Energy
- Reproduction
- Glands

69

Blood Plasma is 90% Water

Sure, blood is thicker than water . . . but only by about 10%! Blood plasma is 90% water which permits it to circulate throughout the body freely. It carries all sorts of nutrients and gases, organic salts and products, and items needed for your bodily functions, activity and growth. Everything used by the body cells is transported by plasma, including the material the cell is made of. Anything made by these same cells which is needed in other parts of the body – or to be excreted – is carried by the same plasma. Yet plasma remains fairly identical in composition at all times throughout the body. As it

---

There is only one water that is clean and that is steam distilled water.
No other substance on our planet does so much to keep us
 healthy and get us well as distilled water does!
– James F. Balch, M.D., author, "Dietary Wellness"

absorbs foods and fuels from the digestive and respiratory processes, it has the same substances taken from it by body tissues, including the kidneys and lungs. If this vital balance is to always be healthy and maintained, it's vitally important to have sufficient pure water for your blood and your entire body.

Water Keeps Us Cool and Healthy

Automobiles have water in their radiators to help cool their engines. It's much the same with the human body. The reason is that water absorbs heat readily. In living organisms, where constant internal temperatures are often critical, water acts as a vital and efficient coolant. The human body has a constant temperature level, measured orally, at 98.6° F. It shouldn't vary much despite the climate or temperature surrounding the body. This internal temperature is controlled by external skin evaporation to a large degree. Just about a fourth of the heat created by the processing of oxygen and food by the body is eliminated through normal perspiration and the process of breathing. But under exceptionally dry conditions, the body can lose up to a quart of water an hour through the sweating process alone. Obviously, this water has to be replaced or other functions of the body are impaired. When it's cold, the body can actually cease perspiring and water is withdrawn into tissues. The evaporation of water from skin surfaces results in cooling – this is Mother Nature's air conditioning and fevers are in a way related. When you sweat and feel hot, perhaps you have a temperature. When your skin is dry and you feel chills, perhaps your body temperature has dipped. These are often signs of an alerting illness.

In humid weather, evaporation is more difficult, so we feel hotter when we're sweating. Our body has a harder time cooling off and ends up working harder to keep it cool. Researchers have found that the average man, doing nothing, will lose about 23 ounces of fluid via the lungs and skin on a day that has normal humidity. A long distance runner, on the other hand, can lose as much as 1-4 pounds an hour. Football players can shed 3% of their body weight of water in an hour's time!

Because the body is more than 75% water (see chart on page 74), and because excretory processes depend so much on it, water is easy to lose. Many so-called diets are based on lower water consumption or increasing water loss. This can be very dangerous! Fatigue is usually the body's first sign of water dehydration. Listen to your body by drinking sufficient water to operate your miracle body machine!

Water is the Body's Vital Miracle Lubricant

The body, in its own way, is greased and oiled automatically. The body's basic lubricant is water. It permits organs to slide against each other – such as when you bend down. It helps the bones to move in their joints. We couldn't bend a knee or elbow without it. It acts as a shock-absorber to ward off injury. Applied hydraulically in various parts of the body, it is used to build and hold pressure. The eyeball is a good example of this particular function of water. Muscle tone cannot be maintained without adequate water, for the muscles are 75% water (see page 74).This is another reason why fatigue hits the dehydrated body. Water flows through every single part of our body, cleansing and nourishing it. But the wrong kind of water – with inorganic minerals, harmful toxins, chemicals and contaminants can pollute and clog our body, gradually stiffening it painfully.

The Body's Three Sources of Water

Your body has to obtain water somehow, to survive. The **first source** is obvious. We drink water or a fluid containing it such as juice, soup, beverages. The **second source** is regular foods, like organic fruits and vegetables which have the highest water content. A peach is almost all water, about 90%. Even something as hard as a dry roll is one quarter water!

Pure water performs miracles internally and externally for well-being.
– Patricia Bragg, Pioneer Health Crusader

"Water contains healing; it is the simplest, cheapest and – if used correctly
– the safest remedy. Water is my best friend and will remain all my life!"
– Father Sebastian Kneipp, Father of Hydrotherapy • www.kneipp.com

The **third source** of important water is metabolism. This is called metabolic water and it's made by the body from raw materials taken into the body. In other words, it's a chemically made water. It results from the cells' conversion of ingested food to cellular food. A perfect example of this type of water production is the biological water factory known as the camel. Now, the camel doesn't store water. It stores fat in the hump on its back. It eats carbohydrates. In using these foods, the camel creates a great deal of water as a by-product and then uses the water in its body chemistry just as if it had drunk the water! Some insects are able to do this too, even though they eat exceptionally dry, low-water content foods. The average man consumes only about 2¹/₂ quarts of water a day by eating and drinking, but he uses to 2³/₄ to 3 quarts. The difference is made up by the production of metabolic water.

Body Dehydration Causes Health Problems

When the body doesn't get enough water, it reacts and suffers! Body dehydration is often called our number one largest health concern. The precious secretions of important glands are drastically deprived when we are dehydrated. Saliva dries up, membranes dry out. We're thirsty. The body signals quickly that a drink of water is imperative! After losing more than a little water without replenishing the supply, other symptoms develop. Headaches, inability to concentrate, nervousness, digestive problems, lack of hunger, all of these are the results of dehydration. Water alleviates all these symptoms. American soldiers in the Arctic experienced personality problems when forced into low-water rations. To be deprived of water for just a few days can be deadly. The body needs 8-10 glasses of water a day to ensure health and survival.

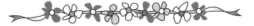

Pure water is the cheapest form of medicine to a dehydrated body.
It is a free investment for your long-term health!
– F. Batmanghelidj, M.D., author of "Your Body's Many Cries for Water"
(You're not sick, you're thirsty, don't treat thirst with medication.)
Please visit website: www.WaterCure.com

Fluoride Is A Deadly Poison!

Millions of innocent people have been brainwashed by aluminum companies to erroneously believe that adding sodium fluoride (their waste by-product) to our drinking water will reduce tooth decay in children. Americans get fluoride in their drinking water without thinking about it. Sodium fluorine, a chemical "cousin" of sodium fluoride, is used as a rat and roach killer and deadly pesticide! Yet this deadly fluoride, injected almost by the government edict into our drinking water in proportion of 1.2 parts per million (PPM), has been declared by the U.S. Public Health Service to be *"safe for all human consumption."* Every chemist knows that such "absolute safety" is not only false and unattainable, but totally an illusion!

We Must Keep Fluoride Out of Our Water and Our Bodies!

Most of the water Americans drink has fluoride in it, including: tap, bottled, canned drinks, soups, and foods! The ADA (American Dental Association) is insisting the FDA (Food and Drug Administration) mandate the addition of fluoride to all bottled waters! Please defend your right to drink pure, non-fluoridated tap and bottled waters! Challenge and stop local and state water fluoridation policies! Please call, write, fax or e-mail the President, your Governor, Senators and state officials (see website: *firstgov.gov*) and send them a copy of the Bragg Water book.

73

CHECK FOLLOWING WEBSITES FOR FLUORIDE UPDATES:

- Fluoride.Mercola.com
- www.FluorideResearch.org
- www.FluorideAlert.org
- www.Fluoridation.com

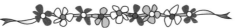

Water is the essential fluid of life – the solvent dissolver of our ills.
Pure water is the deliverer of a radiant, long life.

Distillation effectively removes the widest variety of toxins and contaminants from water. – David and Anne Frähm, authors of "Healthy Habits"

THE 75% WATERY HUMAN

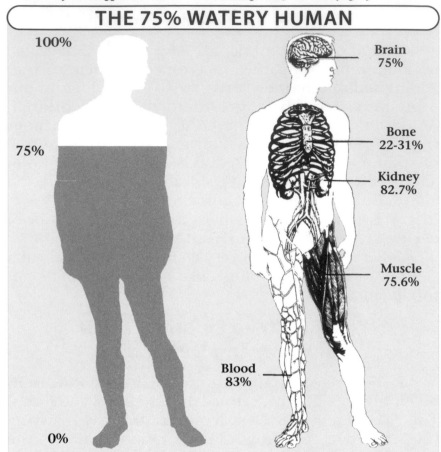

The amount of water in human body, averaging 75%, varies considerably even from one part of the body to another area as shown here. A lean man may hold 75% of his weight in body water, while a woman – because of her larger proportion of adipose tissues – may be only 52% water. The lowering of the water content in the blood is what triggers the hypothalamus, the brain's vital thirst center, to send out its familiar urgent demand for a drink of water! Please obey and drink ample amounts (8 glasses) of purified, distilled water daily. By the time you feel thirsty, you're already dehydrated. – American Running & Fitness Association

WATER PERCENTAGE IN VARIOUS BODY PARTS:

Teeth	10%	Spleen	75.5%
Bones	22-31%	Lungs	80%
Cartilage	55%	Blood	83%
Red blood corpuscles	68.7%	Bile	86%
Liver	71.5%	Plasma	90%
Brain	75%	Lymph	94%
Muscle tissue	75%	Saliva	95.5%

This chart shows why 8-10 glasses of pure water daily is so important.

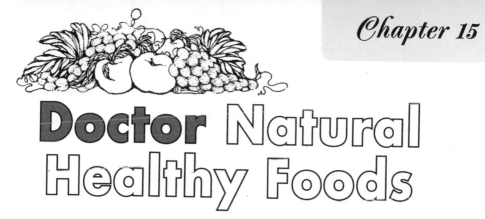

Doctor Natural Healthy Foods

Your body is the most gloriously accurate miracle instrument in this universe! Given the correct fuel, pure air, exercise, sunshine and internal cleansing by fasting, your body will function perfectly and last almost indefinitely! A healthy body is an efficient miracle factory. Given the correct, healthy raw materials, it should be capable (except for accidents) of developing strong healthy tissues and good resistance against most bacteria, viruses and other environmental toxic factors.

It's the only time machine we know of that contains its own repair shop and brain computer! It will work wonders when we give it the proper tools! It's constantly working for us! Biologically, it has no age limit. In fact, there is no biological reason for man to grow old at all. The body has seeds of eternal life! Man doesn't really die, but we commit slow suicide with unhealthy lifestyle habits of living.

Scientists tell us that almost every cell in our body is renewed every 11 months. Then why should anyone worry of being old? Don't believe the old fallacy that as we get older we must face decrepitude, decay, senility and premature death! If people knew what to eat and only ate and lived as they should, *Old Father Time* would shoulder his scythe and walk away!

Most people are suffering from mineral and vitamin deficiencies. Research shows millions are victims of malnutrition and unhealthy lifestyles. The body's millions of red blood cells are constantly dying and being replaced and some are being renewed every second. They can't be rejuvenated properly without the right substances (food nutrients) and these must come from natural, organic, healthy foods (see list pages 120-122).

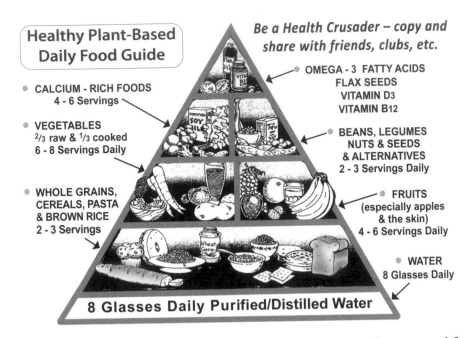

Healthy Plant-Based Daily Food Guide

Be a Health Crusader – copy and share with friends, clubs, etc.

- CALCIUM - RICH FOODS
  4 - 6 Servings

- VEGETABLES
  2/3 raw & 1/3 cooked
  6 - 8 Servings Daily

- WHOLE GRAINS,
  CEREALS, PASTA
  & BROWN RICE
  2 - 3 Servings

- OMEGA - 3 FATTY ACIDS
  FLAX SEEDS
  VITAMIN D3
  VITAMIN B12

- BEANS, LEGUMES
  NUTS & SEEDS
  & ALTERNATIVES
  2 - 3 Servings Daily

- FRUITS
  (especially apples
  & the skin)
  4 - 6 Servings Daily

- WATER
  8 Glasses Daily

8 Glasses Daily Purified/Distilled Water

The Healthy Plant-Based Daily Food Guide Pyramid represents an ideal way of eating for achieving optimal nutrition, health and longevity! You will notice in this Food Guide Pyramid it is based on healthy organic plant-based foods, with an emphasis on fruits, vegetables, whole grains, vegetable protein, non-dairy calcium foods, raw nuts, seeds and purified water. This is the best diet for building a healthy nervous system, disease prevention and to enjoy longevity. Eating a diet based on these dietary guidelines will help the nutrients you need get into your body for optimal health!

At the bottom of the pyramid is **purified water.** We recommend drinking *pure distilled water* as it's the best type of water for the body. At least eight – 8 to 10 oz glasses a day and even more if lifestyle sports, and work require it!

Whole grains are the next pyramid level. Avoid all GMO processed and refined grain products. The next level of the pyramid are **vegetables.** We recommend eating as many of your vegetables organic and raw. On top of that on our pyramid are **fruits.** Fresh, organic fruits!

Life isn't about finding yourself. Life is about creating yourself.
❀ *– George Bernard Shaw, Nobel Prize Winner in Literature, 1925* ❀

Sources of Calcium-Rich Foods

Calcium Food Source	mgs	Calcium Food Source	mgs
Almonds, 1 oz	80	Oatmeal, 1 cup	120
Artichokes, (steamed) 1 cup	51	Orange, 1 large	96
Beans, (white) 1 cup	161	Prunes, 4 whole	45
Bok Choy, (steamed) 1 cup	158	Rhubarb, (cooked) 1 cup	105
Broccoli, (raw/steamed) 1 cup	178	Sesame Seeds, (unhulled) 1 oz	381
Brussel Sprouts, (steamed) 1 cup	56	Soybeans, 1 cup	73
Cabbage, (raw/steamed) 1 cup	50	Soymilk, fortified 1 cup	150
Cauliflower, (raw/steamed) 1 cup	34	Spinach, (raw/steamed) 1 cup	244
Kale, (raw/steamed) 1 cup	180	Tofu, firm 1/2 cup	258
Mustard Greens, 1 cup	138	Turnip greens, 1 cup	198

Sources: *Back to Eden,* Jethro Kloss; *Health Nutrient Bible,* Lynne Sonberg; website: www.vrg.org/nutrition/calcium.htm, chart by Brenda Davis, R.D.

And on top of that rich **calcium foods.** Plant sources of calcium (see chart above) are much healthier than dairy because they don't contain saturated fats or cholesterol. Health calcium-rich foods are tofu, broccoli, green leafy vegetables, etc.

Next on the pyramid are healthy **protein foods.** Vegetable protein foods are more optimal compared to animal protein foods (plant-based protein chart – page 123). They do not contain artery clogging saturated fats and cholesterol. They also contain protective factors to prevent heart disease, cancer and diabetes. Vegetable proteins protect the body and provide it with essential amino acids that it requires. At the top of the pyramid are the **essential nutrients, the essential and healthy fats,** like Omega-3's and Vitamin D. Servings of healthy fats include flaxseed oil, avocado, nuts and seeds and even nutritional yeast. It's wise to provide the body with nutritional supplements that your body requires for health and longevity.

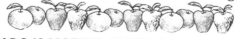

AVOCADO IS MOTHER NATURE'S MIRACLE FOOD:

The avocado tree is strong and requires no spraying with poisonous chemicals. The avocado has perfect balance of life-giving nutrients (potassium, folic acid, fiber, niacin, B6, protein, etc.). It's unsaturated fat helps lower LDL "bad" cholesterol. I eat avocados from our Bragg Organic Farm three times weekly. I mash 3 avocados, add minced garlic, diced onion, juice of 1 lime, chopped cilantro, and a pinch of cayenne pepper. I dip slices of tomato, celery, carrots, apples, cabbage, red onions, cucumbers, bell peppers and lettuce leaves into this "guacamole" for a delicious healthy lunch. – Patricia Bragg

Internal Cleanliness is the Secret of Health

What you want is to strive for a clean, toxin-free body! Gradually include more organic fresh fruits and raw vegetables in your diet. Have fresh fruits in the morning and a large raw, combination vegetable salad at noon. If you like, you may have some fresh fruit for dessert. Eat a yellow vegetable, such as a yam, sweet potato, yellow squash or carrots, and a green vegetable every day.

With your main meal you may have and want a more concentrated form of protein. Our healthiest and favorite proteins are vegetarian! However, if you eat animal proteins, make sure they are organic or wild-caught. You may use natural, cold or expeller pressed oils such as olive, flax, soy, safflower, sunflower and sesame. Read the labels carefully before buying.

Healthy Foods Build and Maintain Your Body!

The person you are today, tomorrow, next week, next month and 10 years from now depends on what you eat! You are the sum total of the food you consume. How you look, feel and carry your years all depends on what you eat! Every part of your body is made from food – the hair on your head, your eyes, teeth, bones, blood and flesh. Even your expression is formed from what you eat, because the healthy man and woman is well-fed and happy. We often jokingly say, "What are we going to feed our faces?" when it is plain that we mean our entire bodies are ready for nourishment.

We can begin anywhere in the body, but it's best starting with the skeleton which supports all other tissues. Superficially, our bones are largely minerals – mostly calcium and phosphate. One might suppose that once the skeleton is formed, nutrition of the bone stops. But this is far from true! Using "isotopic tracers," top biochemists found that, even in an adult body, minerals are constantly leaving and entering the bones. This means that the bones are alive and are dynamic rather than static. Bones contain living cells which require not only minerals, but all the other food nutrients. An emergency need for these cells arises when a bone is broken. If these cells had ceased to live and function when the adult skeleton became formed, a broken bone would remain broken for the rest of our life. When a bone is broken, nourishment of these cells is crucially important! They need not only the minerals required for repairing the damage, but the cells themselves need to "eat" and keep healthy! These bone cells, like all other cells, can be nourished at various levels of efficiency. This is related to the fact that bones sometimes knit slowly and sometimes rapidly! The rate of healing can be slowed dramatically by poor nutrition of the cells, or it can be stepped up by improving the cell's nutrition!

The Whole Body Needs Healthy Foods

Good physicians who treat fracture cases, especially doctors who are nutrition and health-minded make sure that every health measure is taken to promote the finest nutrition possible to mend and build new bone cells!

The cells in our skin, including the hair-building cells, need continual healthy nourishment. This becomes more and more evident when we remember that skin is constantly being shed and replaced, and that hair grows continuously.

Those who handle farm animals, pets or racing animals know that skin and hair sleekness is an important health measurement. If an animal's hair or fur is well-nourished and healthy, it's indication that body cells are nourished. Lab experiments with mammals and fowl show that many entirely different nutritional deficiencies will cause the skin, hair, or feathers, of an animal to become unhealthy. Doctors recognize the appearance of skin and are often able to judge a patient's health condition on the skin alone. Several gross vitamin and mineral deficiencies in humans become obvious by unhealthy skin.

When recovering from accidents or fractures it's important to take extra herbs, mineral and vitamin supplements to nourish and help your body heal faster! – Linda Page, N.D., Ph.D., author "Healthy Healing"

The constipation epidemic is often a manifestation of bad nutrition of the intestinal tissues. There are many "smooth" muscles internally, when stimulated, which cause our stomach and intestinal movements. These wavelike motions called *"peristalsis"* keep the partially digested food moving along until the final residue reaches the large bowel and is eliminated. All these smooth muscles in the colon are made of living cells that must be well nourished. In order to relieve constipation in the intestinal tract, sometimes people will take irritating substances, such as powerful laxatives. These stimulate and drive the muscle cells, sometimes mercilessly, to act when all the muscle cells really need to function is ample liquid and fiber, nutritional habits that are healthy, exercise, fresh air, deep breathing, and a healthy lifestyle.

Iodine from Kelp is Important

80

One of the vital hormones is particularly interesting because it contains a specific chemical element – iodine. The cells that produce the thyroid hormone are among the most differentiated cells in the body . . . they absolutely need iodine to perform their unique function. In certain parts of the world, such as the Great Lakes, the Pacific Northwest and Switzerland, iodine is at a low level in soil and vegetation. As a result, many people have thyroid issues. They become diseased and their thyroid highly swollen, resulting in the condition known as the *"endemic goiter."* They simply cannot do the job of producing the required hormone adequately unless they are furnished with enough iodine to create it. When iodine is furnished from sea vegetation or supplements, the enlarged thyroid gland shrinks to its normal size and problems disappear. By limiting different degrees of iodine in a mammal, it's possible to produce any condition between severe goiter and normal functioning.

The body is self-cleansing, self-correcting and self-healing when you give it a chance with a fasting cleanse and living a healthy lifestyle!
– Patricia Bragg, Pioneer Health Crusader

Healthy Foods Have Good Effect on Brain

At first glance, it appears there is no connection between food and thinking. Yet we assure you, food affects the different parts of the body, and it also affects our thinking! Our thoughts are influenced directly by what we have eaten; especially what we eat habitually.

The brain is given credit for the processes of thought, though some profess to doubt this and maintain that thought originates outside of us, in the ethereal universe. Wherever it originates, the processes are certainly governed by parts of our body. The brain occupies the most strategic position in the body for direction of thoughts and impulses. It is the seat of emotions, motivating impulses and conscious thinking! The brain is the great computer reflex center, from which radiate all nerves that control motion and sensation! Just as the brain depends on blood for fresh oxygen, what we eat determines the health of our blood, our river of life!

Keep Alcohol, Toxins & Drugs Out of Blood!

A brain nourished by blood that is full of toxic poisons is not able to function at its greatest efficiency. Toxins can so befuddle the brain that clear thinking is impossible. Life-threatening comas can result from strong types of intoxication, as in alcohol and drug overdoses.

To have a crystal clear, alert and sharp brain we must keep the toxic poisons in our blood at the lowest possible level. We must eat a diet that will supply all of our brain cells with proper nourishment. Keeping toxic poisons at the lowest level calls for regular fasting and a diet that supplies all the nutrients the brain needs.

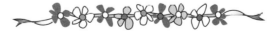

There's no substitute for a healthy diet of organic fruits, vegetables, grains and legumes. Vitamin deficiency usually occurs only after many weeks or months of intake below the recommended daily levels.
– The Complete Guide to Natural Healing

The first wealth is health. – Ralph Waldo Emerson, 1803-1882

Refined, Processed Foods, High in Fat, Salt & Sugar, Produce Learning Disabled Children

To demonstrate the effect that toxic poisons and malnutrition have on children, we have talked to many educators across America. They have thousands of children between the ages of 6 and 17 that are having difficulty being educated. Their brains are slow from toxic poisons and malnutrition because of the Standard American Diet (S.A.D.). These children are being fed breakfast, lunch and dinner foods that are high in fat, salt and sugar. Although the schools are blamed for turning out uneducated students, often this is not the teacher's fault! The blame lies on lifestyle and food choices.

Parents are often misled by TV, radio, magazine and newspaper advertising. This marketing tells the parents to give the child processed foods which are largely composed of refined starch, sugar and fat. These "empty calorie" junk fast foods quickly satisfy a child's appetite, but contain practically no healthy nutrients to build long-term health.

82

America Leads The World in Sickness

America leads the world in the highest standard of living, the largest supplies of food and health care costs! These factors should make it the healthiest nation in the world, not the sickest! And yet it is. America has the gloomiest health forecast and leads the world in degenerative diseases! Why? Maybe because Americans consume more processed, chemicalized, and toxic foods.

Three Needed Health Habits To Enjoy

There are 3 habits which, with but one condition added, will give you everything in the world worth having, beyond which the imagination cannot conjure forth a single added improvement! These habits are:

● **The Health Habit** ● **The Work Habit** ● **The Study Habit**

If you have these habits, and have the love of someone who has these same habits, you are both in paradise! – Elbert Hubbard, 1856-1915

 Learning is a treasure that will follow its owner everywhere. – Chinese Proverb

Enjoy Healthy Fiber for Super Health

These are our suggestions for healthy fiber:

- EAT ALL VARIETIES OF ORGANIC BERRIES, surprisingly good sources of fiber.
- KEEP BEANS HANDY, probably the best fiber sources. Cook dried beans and freeze in portions. Use canned beans for faster meals.
- INSTEAD OF ICEBERG LETTUCE, choose deep green lettuces such as romaine, bib, butter, arugula, spinach, kale, lamb's lettuce or cabbage.
- LOOK FOR "100% ORGANIC WHOLE WHEAT" or whole grain breads, when eating bread.
- LOOK FOR WHOLE GRAIN or RICE CEREALS.
- GO FOR BROWN RICE over white rice.
- EAT THE SKIN of the potato, fruits and vegetables.
- SERVE HUMMUS, made from chickpeas, instead of sour-cream with your dip.
- DON'T UNDERESTIMATE NON-GMO ORGANIC CORN, especially popcorn and corn tortillas.
- ADD ORGANIC OAT BRAN & WHEATGERM to your baked goods.
- SNACK ON ORGANIC SUN-DRIED FRUIT.
- INSTEAD OF DRINKING FRUIT JUICE, eat whole fruit.

– www.BerkeleyWellness.com

Most Common Food Allergies

The most common food allergies are: dairy, cereals and grains, eggs, fish, meats, some fruits – especially citrus fruits, nuts – especially peanuts, chocolate, coffee, cocoa, caffeinated tea, palm and cottonseed oil, and MSG.

Avoid Health-Destroying Habits: Sugar, fat, salt, refined foods and refined flours, chemical preservatives, soda, soft drinks and alcohol.

"We give thanks for unknown blessings already on their way." – Unknown

Warning! – Microwaved Foods Are Unhealthy!

Microwaves have practically replaced traditional cooking, especially in restaurants. But how much do you really know about them? A Swiss Study found food which is microwaved is not the food it was before! The radiation deforms and destroys the molecular structure of the food. For example, microwaving has been found to remove 97% of the flavonoids – plant compounds with anti-inflammatory benefits – in broccoli. That's a third more damage than done by boiling. When microwaved food is eaten, abnormal changes occur in your blood and immune systems! These include a decrease in hemoglobin and white blood cell counts and an increase in cholesterol! An article in the *Pediatrics Journal* warns that microwaving human milk damages the anti-infection properties it usually gives to a mother's baby. Recent work being done at the University of Warwick in Great Britain warns that microwave radiation is damaging to vital electromagnetic activity of human life vibrations.

Beware of Deadly Aspartame and Other Sugar Substitutes

Although it sounds "tame," this deadly neurotoxin Aspartame is anything but! Aspartame is an artificial sweetener (over 200 times sweeter than sugar) made by Monsanto and marketed as "NutraSweet," "Equal," "Spoonful," and countless other trade names. Although aspartame is added to over 9,000 food products, it is not fit for human consumption! This toxic poison changes into formaldehyde in the body and has been linked to migraines, seizures, vision loss and symptoms relating to lupus, Parkinson's, Multiple Sclerosis and many other health destroying conditions. For more information on this toxic killer – please go to: *aspartame.mercola.com*

ASPARTAME – ARTIFICIAL DIET SWEETENER THAT MAKES YOU FAT!
Besides being a deadly poison (see above box), aspartame contributes to weight gain by causing a craving for carbohydrates. A study of 80,000 women by American Cancer Society found those who used this neurotoxic "diet" sweetener actually gained more weight than those who didn't use aspartame products. Some studies also suggest that artificial sweeteners increase appetite, which may promote weight gain. Stevia is a healthier alternative for diabetics.

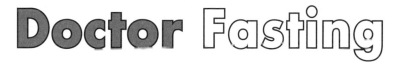
Doctor Fasting

Fasting is accepted and recognized as being the oldest form of therapy. It is mentioned 74 times in the Bible. It is the universal therapy even used by sick animals in the wilds the world over. As we study the ancient healers of the world, we find that fasting heads the list for helping Mother Nature heal the sick and the wounded.

There is a misconception about fasting that must be clarified. It must be definitely and positively stated that fasting is not a cure for any disease or ailment. The purpose of a fast is to allow the body's Vital Force full range and scope to fulfill its own self-healing, self-repairing and self-rejuvenating functions to the best advantage. Healing is an internal biological function. Fasting gives the body a physiological rest and permits the body to become 100% more efficient in healing itself. Fasting under proper care or with workable knowledge is probably the fastest way and safest means of regaining health ever conceived by the human mind!

85

We want to make it clear and positive that fasting does not cure anything. Fasting puts the body in a condition where all the Vital Force of the body is used to flush out the causes of body miseries. **Fasting helps the body help itself.** We who have made a life study of the Science of Fasting and conducted and supervised thousands of fasts know the miracles that the body itself can perform during the period of complete abstinence from solid food. It gives the overworked and overburdened internal organs ample rest and time for rehabilitation! It enhances the internal power and vitality of the body to flush out toxic poisons and wastes that have been stored in the body for years.

    Fasting is Mother Nature's Miracle –
it cleanses, renews and rejuvenates!

Fasting is the greatest remedy, the physician within.
– Paracelsus, 15th Century Physician, Father of Body Chemistry

Fasting raises the Vital Force to its highest efficiency. It promotes the elimination of inorganic chemical accumulations, toxins and other pollutants that cannot be flushed from the body by any other means.

Prophets wisely fasted for spiritual enlightenment and a closer contact with the Divine. We know that fasting sharpens and hones the mental faculties to a keen edge. Fasting improves the organs of mastication, digestion, assimilation and the elimination of food. The mighty liver – which is known as the chemical laboratory of the human body and is typically the most abused organ – at last has a chance during the fast to rehabilitate and gain Vital Force. Thus, after a fast, the liver functions more efficiently. Especially all the sensory powers possessed by the fasting human beings are exhilarated and naturally raised to a higher efficiency level than normal during and after the fast! You can prove this to yourself with your own fast!

86

No process or health therapy ever fulfilled so many indications for restoration of vigorous health as fasting! It's Mother Nature's own prime process and her very first requirement in nearly all cases. After a fast the circulation is better, food can be assimilated, and endurance, stamina and strength are increased! After a fast the mind becomes more alert and receptive to logic and living a wise, sensible, naturally healthy life.

After the fast the mind becomes so powerful that it can take full control of the body. It becomes the complete master and, if a person does not go back to old habits, they can maintain this mastery of the body for the rest of their lives. Fasting instills personal confidence. It gives a person a positive mental attitude and it promotes tranquility of mind and a glow of well-being that no other therapy can offer. Fasting rejuvenates, revives and purifies every one of the trillions of cells that make up the body. *Fasting is the road to internal purity!*

Actress Cloris Leachman – an ardent Bragg health follower sparkled with health. She disliked smoking, coffee, alcohol, sugar and meat.
A solution to any health problem she said is to fast!
"Fasting is a miracle; it cured my years of asthma."

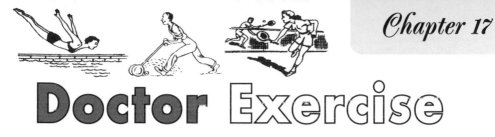

Chapter 17

Doctor Exercise

Doctor Exercise makes this statement, *"To rest is to rust!"* Rust means decay and destruction. In other words, the good doctor tells us that activity is life and stagnation is death. **Activity is the law of life! It is the law of well-being! Every vital organ of the body has its specialized work, and its performance depends on its development, strength and health.**

With exercise, you bring on healthy perspiration. Impurities and toxins are expelled when you exercise and perspire freely – you are allowing the skin to perform its normal function of eliminating poisons. If you don't exercise daily to the point of perspiring, the work that the pores are not doing throws a double burden on the other eliminative organs and then we get into health problems.

When we would stride along on our daily 3-4 mile brisk walk that helped us maintain healthier hearts, bodies and kept our bones strong, we would say to ourselves and often out loud, *'Health, Strength, Youth, Vitality, Joy, Peace and Salvation for Eternity!'*

Start the 10 Minute Trick – It Works Miracles

The successful student of *The Bragg Healthy Lifestyle*, and anyone who has made healthy exercise part of their daily routine, will tell you the same thing: the moment of beginning is the most difficult. The in-between moment after you decide you want to become healthier and before you begin to act on that decision is the hardest moment. The moment before you put that one leg in front of the other on that first step of your brisk walk is the most difficult moment of exercise.

The people who tell you the success stories of exercise recommend "tricking yourself" into exercise at first. Play the "10 minute trick". Before you start (which is the hardest moment), tell yourself, *"I'll only exercise or walk for 10 minutes and then I'll stop. That will be easy and I'll be done soon."* Once you've done this, you're on your path to healthy fitness – and it will get fun! Once this most difficult moment is over (the beginning) you'll find that when the 10 minute mark comes around you are enjoying yourself so much that you won't want to quit!

Exercise Helps Normalize Blood Pressure

Exercise helps to normalize blood pressure and create a healthy pulse. Exercise is an anticoagulant, meaning that it keeps the blood flowing smoothly and not clotting (called a "thrombus" which could cause a heart attack).

Every creature seeking to eliminate internal waste does so by means of muscular action. Inside your intestines there are three muscular layers which undergo a miraculous rhythmic, wavelike action called peristalsis. A serious condition results if you allow internal and external muscles, through inactivity, to just become flabby instead of muscular. The muscles lose their tone and power to contract, resulting in intestinal clogging. The muscles play an important role in the evacuation effort. What happens when the internal and external muscles become soft, sick and infiltrated with fat? They refuse to work and we pile up intestinal waste. This brings about the autointoxication, the building up of large amounts of toxic poisons inside the body. Inactivity is the avoidable cause of so many diseases.

Fasting and diet are two allies in your struggle for long lasting youth, health and symmetry. When it comes to fighting fat, diet and fasting come first. But when it comes to keeping fit, it is exercise that matters most! However, they all help each other, for by exercising regularly you may be more generous in your diet and, up to a certain point, your extra food will just make for increased vitality. The human machine loves exercise, outdoor activities, and it can work at top performance when fit and healthy. As with all machines, it improves with use. Nothing betrays its weak spots like inactivity and rust.

 While exercise is good for the body, it's also good for mental and emotional health.

Brisk Walking For Health, Fitness & Longevity

We believe in all forms of exercise, but without hesitation we will tell you that brisk walking is the best all-around exercise! Of all the forms of exercise, walking brings most of the body into healthy action!

No other exercise gives the same body harmony of movement and improved circulation. Brisk walking is the best exercise for almost everyone. Let it be fun and natural. Walk tall with your head high, spine and chest lifted up! You will feel elated, so you will carry yourself proudly, straight, erect and with arms swinging. It's fun to have a *Flex™ Heart Monitor* – a wireless activity and sleep wristband device. This will keep track of your walking distance and it can even wake you silently in the morning. It's the motivation you need to get walking and be more active! See web: *FitBit.com*

Vow to become a health walker and make your daily brisk walk a fixed item in your health program all year. Stride with your spirit free. If the outer world of nature fails to interest you, turn to the inner world of the mind. As you walk, your body ceases to matter and you become a near poet and philosopher as you will ever be. **Walking has astounding miracles for your health! A study published in the *New England Journal of Medicine* shows that walking 30 minutes a day, three times a week, reduces risk of death from all natural causes by 55%! Research shows walking releases pent-up emotions, like anger and frustration, and reduces stress, tension and depression.**

It's never too late to start exercising! Studies show that recent physical activity has a greater positive impact on cardiovascular disease and mortality than exercise done in one's past. The cardiovascular health benefits of recent physical activity are more pronounced than with distant physical activity, even though both are beneficial. A consistent maintenance exercise program produces the best overall results!
– Sports Medicine Digest – See web: TheSportDigest.com

Progress is impossible without change, and those who cannot change their minds, cannot change anything. – George Bernard Shaw, 1880's

Gardening is another rewarding form of exercise! But gardening may not prevent weight gain if there is too little movement, because you are bent over instead of being erect. For this reason, we prefer both. Satisfy your conscience by applying your energy productively in your healthy garden, and then take the kink out of your back with a brisk walk. In our personal life, we combine gardening with calisthenics, rebounding (trampoline), brisk walking, weightlifting, swimming, and tennis.

The Importance of Abdominal Exercises

We believe that the most important exercises are those that stimulate all of the muscles of the human trunk from the hips to the armpits. These are the binding muscles which hold all the vital organs in place. When you develop your torso's muscles, also called your core, you are also developing your internal muscles and your posture! As your back, waist, chest and abdomen increase in strength and elasticity, so will your lungs, heart, stomach, and kidneys, gain in efficiency.

The more you fast – the more toxins and fat you will clean from your body! As your body increases in internal cleanliness, your muscles will have more tone and vitality. You will find after a fast that the old sluggish, feelings are gone, replaced with a desire for more exercise and physical activity. And you will bubble with new found energy.

Should You Exercise While Fasting?

This is a question that only you can answer. If there is no inclination for physical activity during a fast, then you should not exercise. The fast is giving you a physiological rest and – unless you have a tremendous, urge for physical activity – it is wise to rest and relax. Your body is using all of its Vital Force for internal purification. But if you feel that you need some stretching or walking during a 7-to 10-day fast, by all means enjoy it. It's between fasts and in your daily *Bragg Healthy Lifestyle* that you should spend a portion of each day of your life pursuing outdoor exercise, walking, or gardening, whenever possible.

Iron Pumping Oldsters (ages 86 to 96) Triple Muscle Strength in U.S. Government Study

A group of frail Boston nursing home residents, aged 86 to 96, turned into weight-lifters to demonstrate that it is never too late to reverse age-related declines in muscle strength. This group participated in a regimen of high-intensity weight-training in a study conducted by the Agriculture Department's Human Nutrition Research Center on Ageing at Tufts University in Boston. *"A high-intensity weight-training program is capable of inducing dramatic increases in muscle strength in frail men and women up to 96 years of age,"* reported the study director, a dedicated researcher, Dr. Maria A. Fiatarone.

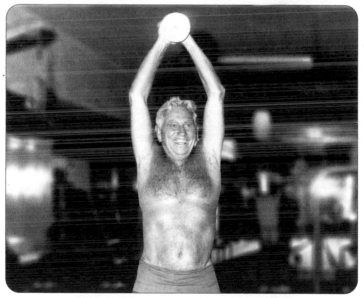

Paul C. Bragg lifting weights.

Paul would practice progressive weight training 3 times a week to stay healthy and fit. Scientists have proven weight training works miracles for all ages by maintaining more flexibility, energy and youthful stamina!

Brisk walking performs physical, mental and spiritual miracles and wards off diseases, reduces stress and improves heart health, circulation, helps normalize weight, blood pressure and cholesterol.
– PBS T.V. Mark Fenton, author, "Pedometer Walking: Stepping Your Way to Health, Weight Loss and Fitness."

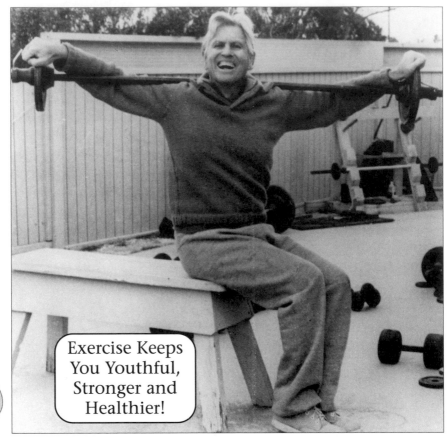

Exercise Keeps
You Youthful,
Stronger and
Healthier!

Paul C. Bragg and Patricia lifted weights three times weekly.

Amazing Health & Fitness Results in 8 Weeks

"The favorable response to strength training in our subjects" she said, "was remarkable in light of their advanced ages, sedentary habits, multiple chronic diseases, functional disabilities and nutritional inadequacies. The elderly weight-lifters increased their muscle strength by anywhere from three to four-fold in as little as eight weeks." **Dr. Fiatarone said that many were stronger at the end of the program than they had been in years!**

To insure good health: exercise, eat lightly, breathe deeply,
live moderately, cultivate cheerfulness and
maintain an interest in life. – William Louden

Exercise, deep breathing, healthy foods, with some fasting helps
maintain a healthier physical balance for a longer, happier life!

Dr. Fiatarone and associates emphasized the safety of such a closely supervised weight-lifting program, even among people in frail health. The average age of the ten participants was 90. Six had coronary heart disease; seven had arthritis; six had bone fractures resulting from osteoporosis; four had high blood pressure; and all had been physically inactive for years. Yet, no serious medical complications resulted from the weight-training, only positive health outcomes!

Muscle atrophy and muscle weakness are not merely cosmetic problems in elderly people, especially the frail elderly. Researchers have linked muscle weakness with recurrent falls, a major cause of immobility and death in the American elderly population. This results in millions of dollars yearly in staggering medical costs.

Previous studies have suggested that weight-training can be helpful in reversing age-related muscle weakness. Dr. Fiatarone said physicians have been reluctant to recommend weight-lifting for frail elderly people with multiple health problems. The United States government study might change their minds. Also, this study shows the great importance in keeping the 640 muscles in our body as active and fit as possible to maintain general overall good health!

93

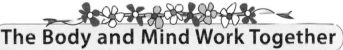

The Body and Mind Work Together

Whatever occurs in the mind affects the body and vice versa. The mind and the body cannot be considered independently. When the two are out of sync, then both emotional and physical stress can erupt.
– Hippocrates, The Father of Medicine

The body is the soul's house. Shouldn't we take care of our house so it doesn't fall into ruin?
– Philo of Alexandria, wise philosopher, 20 B.C.

Miracles can happen daily through guidance and prayer!
– Patricia Bragg

Time waits for no one, treasure and protect every moment you have!

Do These Exercises Daily (10 per set):

You must exercise, for weak muscles of the arms, legs and entire body indicates a similar condition of the stomach muscles and the other body organs.

Important exercises for keeping the external and internal trunk muscles of the stomach fit and healthy. These exercises also promote good elimination.

Bend at the waist to the sides, then front and back.

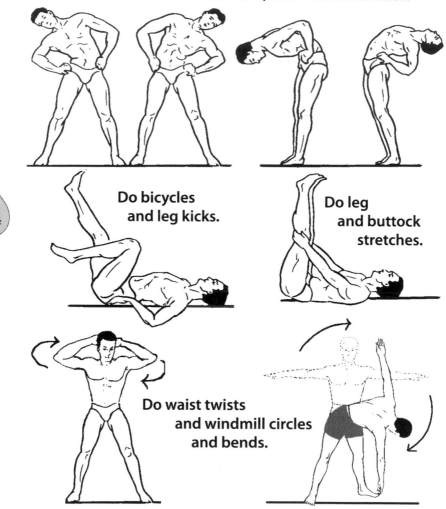

Do bicycles and leg kicks.

Do leg and buttock stretches.

Do waist twists and windmill circles and bends.

94

Exercise, with fasting and The Bragg Healthy Lifestyle, helps cleanse, restore and maintain a healthy physical balance in your daily living for a long, happy life. – Paul C. Bragg, N.D., Ph.D., Pioneer Health Crusader

❀ ❀ *Wise, faithful fasting and exercise aids in* ❀ ❀
preventing excess body weight for maintaining a healthy, fit body!

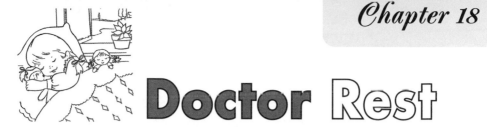

Chapter 18

Doctor Rest

Doctor Rest is another specialist who is always at your command to help you win Supreme Vitality. We believe the word "rest" is the most misunderstood word in the dictionary. Some people's idea of resting is to sit down and drink a cup coffee or tea or a soft drink. This is particularly evident in the modern coffee break for employees. But rest means to repose . . . freedom from activity . . . quiet and tranquility. It means peace of mind and spirit. It means to rest without anxiety or worry. It means to refresh oneself. Your rest should refresh your whole nervous system and your entire body.

It does not mean sitting with one leg crossed over the other. When we sit with our legs crossed we are putting a tremendous burden on the artery which supplies blood to the knee joint and muscles of the leg and foot. You also cut off nerve energy. So if you sit with one leg crossed over the other leg, you are not resting – you are giving the heart a tremendous load of work to do! Don't cross your legs when you sit down – keep both feet on the floor (see page 103).

To properly rest and be still, it's also important to wear no restricting garments that might hinder your blood circulation. Are your shoes too tight? Your collar? Your hat? Your belt? Your watch? Your stockings? If so, then you are not really resting when you sit still or lie down. The best rest is secured when you have loose or very little clothing on. Any clothes and shoes you are wearing should be comfortably loose and never binding!

Help me to know the magical restoring power of sleep. – Hittite Prayer

Nothing in all creation is so like God as stillness. – Meister Eckhart

The average person spends about 24 years of a 78 year lifespan asleep.

You cannot attain healthy relaxation in the true sense of the word when you use toxic stimulants and nerve destroying drugs.

CHECK YOUR MATTRESS

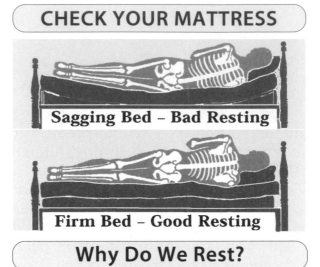

Sagging Bed – Bad Resting

Firm Bed – Good Resting

Why Do We Rest?

Another form of rest is to take a short nap. When taking naps, you command your muscles to become completely relaxed. Sleep is the great revitalizer, but so few people get a long, peaceful and refreshing night's sleep. Many people use stimulants: tobacco, drugs, coffee, tea, alcohol, sugar, and cola drinks. All of these whip the tired nerves, so when you use these stimulants you can never have complete rest and relaxation.

96

Rest and Sleep Must Be Earned

A body full of toxins is a constant irritant to the nerves. How is it possible to get a good night's rest with irritated nerves? It's not. In our years of experience with fasting we have found that when people discard stimulants when fasting, they become deep, restful sleepers! You will notice as you purify your body that you will be able to relax more deeply. You will be able to enjoy naps and the benefits of a recharging and good night's sleep.

For sleep problems try melatonin, calcium, magnesium, valerian capsules and extracts, 5-HTP tryptophan, Sleepytime Tea and valerian herbal teas.

Nervous Tension can ruin your health in dozens of ways and diminish your productivity and even shorten your lifespan.
– Dr. Edmund Jacobson, author, "You Must Relax"

Mother Nature Knows What's Best!

One of the predominant suggestions of this book is a gradual return to Mother Nature and her way of natural living. In food, clothing, rest, sleep and simplicity in living habits, try to reach a nearness to Mother Nature that makes you almost one with her. When you feel that the same pure forces that express themselves in a beautiful pine tree are expressing themselves in you, you have made a big stride toward a healthy ideal.

Begin to live as wise Mother Nature wants you to live. Seek to feel that she claims you and you are part of all healthy, growing things. Put yourself into her hands and let her guide you! You will rekindle your own youth in the quiet beauty of the hill and the meadow. If you are to grow more healthy and youthful, begin by believing you can and that Mother Nature is eager to aid you! Better than any human or divine agency, Mother Nature can support your body and your mind and redeem you to health. If you are a prisoner of the city, make it a point to get out to the parks or country or the seashore where you can really find true rest, tranquility and serenity.

97

In a loving way, we have tried to stress these points. Faithfully demand of yourself a higher standard of superb health and happiness. We cannot receive higher health unless our body gets its rest periods to develop new vitality and energy. Second, regard your priceless body as a miracle machine under your care and control! Every machine must have rest periods! If not, you will build up too much friction. That's what so many Americans do in their busy lives, and that creates nerve irritation. Third, with increasing years, draw closer and more intimately to Mother Nature. You should cease to look for thrills and over-stimulation; instead, seek a peaceful life! By living in simplicity and purity, you will be filled with peace, joy and love.

Humor is healthy – it improves blood circulation, boosts immune system, and helps relieve stress. – Dr. Joel Goodman, "Laffirmations"

How beautiful a day can be when kindness touches it.
– George Elliston

Relax and Enjoy Your Life – It's No Crime

Let health, air, sun and complete rest work for you. With a serene clear eye and confidence, put yourself in Mother Nature's hands. Let her run your machine, heal your hurts and comfort you in sickness and adversity. Then, when you have lived a long life of usefulness and happiness, let her call you home. Make Mother Nature your partner and – when you are resting, relaxing, and recreating new energy – she will always be there with a loving hand on your shoulder. Be a child of Mother Nature.

In America we are prone to look down on the person who wants to relax or live a leisurely life – they are so often called lazy. It seems we must be doing something every moment. We must be busy talking, listening to music, watching TV, working. We have parties to attend, athletic events and programs of all kinds. We are constantly pushing and driving our bodies and minds. No wonder so many people have emotional problems. Even psychiatrists and psychologists are overworked. Americans tend to rush and keep too busy! Please don't be ashamed to relax and get off the treadmill. At times it's fun to do nothing, it's healthful and necessary.

You have a natural, built-in tranquilizer located in the muscle cells. Don't expect to use sedatives, become skilled in healthy relaxation. We have known people who discarded their sedatives after becoming fasters and employing Mother Nature as their guardian in life.

Tips for Healthful Sound Sleep

- Avoid and don't use stimulants such as caffeine (found in coffee, tea, cola drinks) and nicotine (found in all tobacco products).
- Don't drink alcohol to "help" you sleep, it disturbs normal sleep patterns.
- Exercise regularly. Get gentle sunshine. Finish workout 2-3 hours before bedtime. Yoga and stretching quiets the mind and body.
- Establish regular, relaxing bedtime routine. For example, try a relaxing aromatherapy or warm vinegar bath or shower.
- Associate your bed with relaxing sleep – don't use it to work or watch TV. Keep sleep area quiet & dark (use ear plugs & eye shade if needed).
- If you suffer from insomnia, don't take naps until problem is corrected.

Chapter 19

Doctor Good Posture

PERFECT POSTURE AND ALIGNMENT

Why should emphasis be placed on resisting the pull of gravity? This is easy to explain. In the past, as long as your muscles were strong enough they held up your skeleton – with its many points and sections – in proper balance and free from strain or discomfort. Maybe now your muscles are losing the battle with gravity. Maybe you have become prematurely older, heavier or inactivity has weakened your muscles just enough to cause you pain and an uncomfortable state of balance causing poor posture.

Such sagging stretches the ligaments of your back and can cause backaches. Ligaments that are unduly stretched are painful. Your ligaments are meant to serve only as stops for the joints and they cannot be forcibly stretched without pain. When the ligaments in your back are made uncomfortable by stretching, it is only natural for your muscles to try to oppose the down sagging of your back which results from the pull of gravity.

99

When your muscles are too weak to do their proper job, they rapidly become exhausted and develop the terrible misery of fatigue, making your back even more uncomfortable! Do you notice a deep aching and soreness along the spine from stretched ligaments? Are your back and shoulders achy and tired? Is your backache basically due to weak muscles? If it is, you can do something sensible to relieve it, and enjoy strengthening those weak muscles with proper exercise.

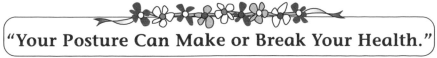

"Your Posture Can Make or Break Your Health."

Take the Mirror Posture Test

Look at yourself in the mirror. Do your shoulders slump? Is your upper back round? Are you a swayback? The bending, slumping, ligament-stretching force of gravity has taken its toll. But even if you are presently a sufferer of backache due to weak muscles and bad posture, don't despair. You can restore back comfort with this posture exercise (see below) and *The Bragg Healthy Lifestyle.*

It has often been said that backache is the penalty man must pay for the privilege of walking and standing upright on two feet, often wearing uncomfortable shoes. Every infant struggles to stand instinctively on his own two feet and walk. He need not be taught. He will attempt this bipedal gait even if left alone most of the time and never instructed. It is natural for a human being to stand and walk in this manner. This is interesting, because there are no animals which spend all of their standing and walking hours on two feet, not even gorillas or chimpanzees. These apes use their hands and arms to help them move about. The world's strongest gorilla would be unable to follow a busy person, walking erectly, for more than a short time. This is because human beings are meant to walk erect!!! and animals are not!

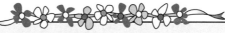

Bragg Posture Exercise Gives Instant Youthfulness

Before a mirror, stand up, feet 8" apart, stretch up your spine. Tighten your buttocks and suck in your stomach muscles, lift up the rib cage, put the chest out, shoulders back, and chin up slightly. Line the body up straight, drop hands to the sides and swing your arms to normalize posture. Do this posture exercise daily and miraculous changes will happen! You are retraining and strengthening your muscles to stand straight for health and youthfulness. Remember when you slump, you also cramp your precious machinery. This posture exercise will retrain your frame to sit, stand and walk tall for supreme health, and longevity!

Whatever occurs in the mind, affects the body and visa versa.
Mind and body cannot be considered independently. When the two
are out of sync, both the emotional and physical stress can erupt.
– Hippocrates, the Father of Medicine, 400 B.C.

Remember – Your posture can make or break your looks and health!

Good Posture Important For Health & Looks

The spines of human beings have natural curves which enable the muscles to oppose gravity and hold their backs erect. As long as the muscles are strong and able to maintain the balance of these curves the back is comfortable. When the muscles are weak, the back sags, ligaments are stretched and that causes backaches.

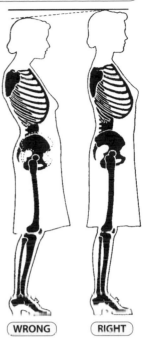

WRONG   RIGHT

To maintain oneself in a healthy state involves many factors: natural foods, rest, sleep, fasting, controlling our emotions and mind and, last but not least, good posture. If the body is properly health nourished and cared for, good posture is not a problem. When the body lacks the essentials, poor posture is often the result. Once poor habits have been established, we must faithfully each day practice corrective exercises and good posture habits.

How to Sit, Stand and Walk
For Strength, Health and Youthfulness

When walking, one should imagine that the legs are attached to the middle of the chest. This gives long, sweeping, graceful, springy steps because, when one walks correctly with this swing and spring, he then automatically builds energy. Habit either makes or breaks us, and good posture habits make graceful, strong bodies. Just as the twig is bent, the tree is inclined.

When in a sitting position, see that the spine is stretched up and backed against the chair. Put shoulders back and lift your chest up and off the stomach, head high and never forward. Be sure to have both your feet on the floor and never sit with your legs crossed! Under the knees run two of the largest arteries, carrying nourishing blood to the muscles below the knees and to all the important nerves that are found in the feet.

WHERE DO YOU STAND?

POSTURE CHART

	PERFECT	FAIR	POOR
HEAD			
SHOULDERS			
SPINE			
HIPS			
ANKLES			
NECK			
UPPER BACK			
TRUNK			
ABDOMEN			
LOWER BACK			

102

Your posture carries you through life from your head to your feet.
This is your human vehicle and you are truly a miracle! Cherish, respect
and protect it by living The Bragg Healthy Lifestyle. – Patricia Bragg

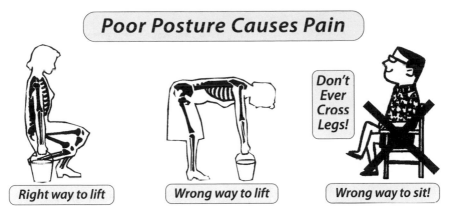

Poor Posture Causes Pain

Don't Ever Cross Legs!

Right way to lift

Wrong way to lift

Wrong way to sit!

When you cross your legs you immediately cut down the flow of blood to almost a trickle. When the leg and knee muscles are not nourished and don't have good circulation, the blood goes stagnant in the extremities which can lead to varicose veins and broken capillaries. Look at the ankles of people over 40 who have made it a habit of crossing their legs and you will see broken veins and capillaries. When the muscles and feet don't get their full supply of blood, the feet become weak and poor circulation sets in. Cold feet torment leg-crossers.

A well known heart specialist was once asked, "When do most people have a heart attack?" The heart specialist answered, "At a time they are sitting quietly with one leg crossed over the other." So you can see that when you sit down, you should plant both of your feet squarely on the floor. People who are habitual leg-crossers always have more acid crystals stored in the feet than those who never cross their legs while sitting. Crossing of the legs is one of the worst postural habits of mankind! It throws the hips, spine and the head off balance and can become one of the most insidious causes of a chronic backache. Poor posture of any kind can bring unbearable pain especially in the neck and lower back.

One very simple habit that is very beneficial to establish for your health is to stand, walk and sit tall and never sit with your legs crossed! Good posture does not require an exaggerated unhealthy position. It's simply stretching up your spine and standing erect – which gives all your body's machinery room to operate and keep you healthier!

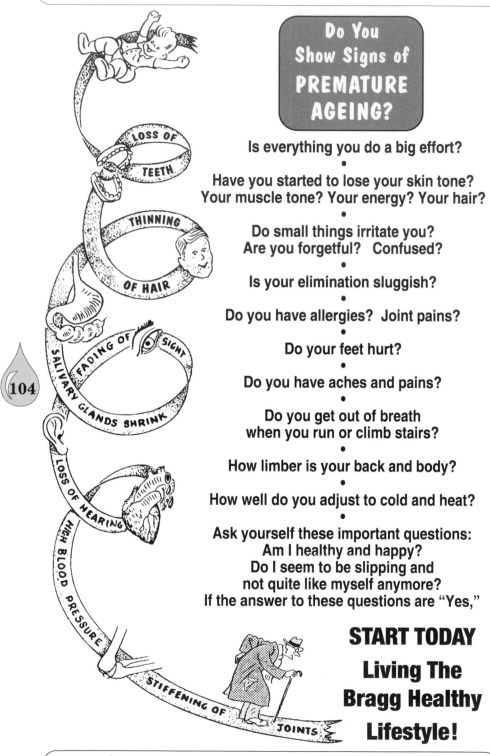

Do You Show Signs of PREMATURE AGEING?

Is everything you do a big effort?

•

Have you started to lose your skin tone?
Your muscle tone? Your energy? Your hair?

•

Do small things irritate you?
Are you forgetful?   Confused?

•

Is your elimination sluggish?

•

Do you have allergies? Joint pains?

•

Do your feet hurt?

•

Do you have aches and pains?

•

Do you get out of breath
when you run or climb stairs?

•

How limber is your back and body?

•

How well do you adjust to cold and heat?

•

Ask yourself these important questions:
Am I healthy and happy?
Do I seem to be slipping and
not quite like myself anymore?
If the answer to these questions are "Yes,"

START TODAY

Living The

Bragg Healthy

Lifestyle!

LOSS OF TEETH

THINNING OF HAIR

FADING OF SIGHT

SALIVARY GLANDS SHRINK

LOSS OF HEARING

HIGH BLOOD PRESSURE

STIFFENING OF JOINTS

104

He who understands nature walks with God. – Edgar Cayce

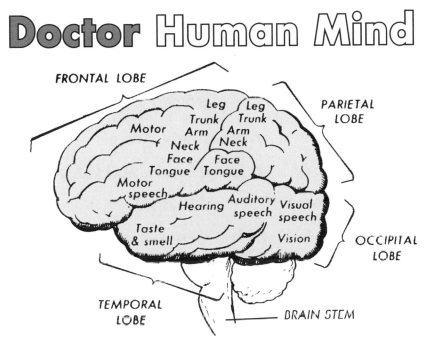

Chapter 20

Doctor Human Mind

FRONTAL LOBE

PARIETAL LOBE

Leg / Leg
Trunk / Trunk
Motor Arm / Arm
Neck / Neck
Face / Face
Tongue / Tongue
Motor speech
Hearing Auditory speech Visual speech
Taste & smell
Vision

OCCIPITAL LOBE

TEMPORAL LOBE

BRAIN STEM

A Healthy Mind in a Healthy Body

What has your mind to do with health and long life? **105** Think of your thoughts as powerful magnets, as entities which have the ability to attract or repel, according to how they are used! A majority of people lean either to the positive or the negative side mentally. The positive phase is constructive and goes for success and positive achievements, while the negative side of life is destructive, leading to futility and failure. It's self-evident that it's to our advantage to cultivate a positive healthy mental attitude. With patience, persistence and living *The Bragg Healthy Lifestyle* this can easily be accomplished.

There are many negative and destructive forms of thought which react in every cell in your body. The strongest are fear and worry – along with depression, anxiety, apprehension, jealousy, envy, anger, and self-pity. All of these negative thoughts bring tension

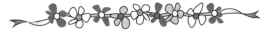

Please be a good, wise, strict, loving, Mother-like Captain to your Miracle Working Body that is carrying you through life!
– Patricia Bragg, Pioneer Health Crusader and Life Coach

to the body and mind leading to energy depravation and a slow or rapid poisoning of the body! Worry and other destructive emotions act slowly but, in the end, can have the same destructive effect as toxic food. Anger and intense fear stop the digestive action, upset the kidneys and the colon, and can cause total body upheaval. Fear, worry and other destructive habits of thought can muddle the mind! A crystal clear mind is needed to reason to your best advantage.

Let Your Mind Guide You to Health!

In your mind, form an image of the person you want to be. Now, with Mother Nature's Nine Doctors as your helpers, you can make yourself into exactly what you want to be! Believe in the power of positive thinking! Practice thought substitution. Never let a negative thought take over your mind! In this way, you set your own pattern of living and you make your mind a powerhouse of positive thoughts.

Mind-Soul-Body Miracle Rewards with Fasting:

- Each time you fast, your mind becomes stronger, healthier and more positive and peaceful.
- Each time you fast, you will continue to eliminate fear, worry and negative emotions and habits.
- Fasting elevates the soul, the mind and the body. What greater miracle rewards can you desire in life?

By fasting, you can create the person you have always desired to be. That is, you can if you faithfully pursue and seek the best that life can offer! When the body and mind are in harmony there will be opportunity for proper spiritual and mental development. Never forget that the spiritual man comes first, the mental is second and the physical third. When the second and third aspects are in harmony there will be a proper balanced, beautiful, peaceful and spiritual life!

Ten Little, Two-Letter Words of Action To Say Daily:
"If it is to be, it is up to me!"

Chapter 21

Spiritual Aspects of Fasting

As a Health Crusader for the many miraculous benefits of fasting for over 70 years, it's gratifying to see the increased interest among scientists that's developed these last decades. Not only have health professionals rediscovered fasting as Mother Nature's primary method of healing and preventing sickness, but churches are awakening to the importance of fasting for spiritual growth.

We are faithful in following our fasting as outlined in this book. That is one of the reasons for our long, healthy life! We are blessed to see the fruition of our world health outreach to help make the world healthier.

During the first three quarters of the 20th century, we saw the world becoming more complex, chaotic and unhealthy. Most humans were feeling alienated, lost and confused.

In time of deep trouble, our natural instincts lead us back to the fundamentals of Mother Nature's Natural Laws. This return is usually made with knowledge gained from hard-learned lessons. Fasting as the means of purifying and healing the body, mind and spirit is instinctive with animals, infants and among many cultures. Now we are beginning to learn the power of this simple, natural method. Many books and articles are appearing that show the spiritual and physical benefits of fasting.

107

Fasting Gives Mental & Physical Awareness

As the body cleanses and heals itself through fasting, keener mental concentration and clearer spiritual perception develop. Remember, the brain is the physical instrument of the mind. As the mucus and toxic wastes are flushed from the brain cells, with that go worries and frustrations from your mind. Your mind will become free and clear. You are thinking intelligently and logically. Your memory will become sharp and keen. Your creative powers will expand. You will be able to face reality and yourself . . . and begin to view your problems objectively to find definite answers – and solutions!

The elimination of toxic wastes releases the mind from physical bondage. The freedom from the bodily necessity of procuring, preparing, eating, digesting and assimilating food frees up and releases a tremendous amount of nervous energy which invigorates the mental and spiritual processes. You attain new levels of tranquility, serenity and peace of mind. You become spiritually perceptive and receptive and at one with the Infinite.

Great Spiritual Leaders Practiced Fasting

The founders of the modern world's four major religions – Christianity, Judaism, Buddhism and Islam – taught fasting as a means of communication with the Divine through purification of body, mind and spirit. They instructed fasting should be carried out with dedication and in private. Similar teachings are found in nearly all religions, ancient and tribal, as well as influential philosophies and moral codes. Zoroaster, the great Persian prophet, taught and practiced fasting. So did Plato, Socrates and Aristotle. Hippocrates, the Father of Medicine, considered fasting the great cleanser and healer. The genius painter and sculptor Leonardo da Vinci also practiced and advocated fasting.

China's great philosopher and teacher, Confucius, included fasting in all his precepts. The Yogis of India and Native Americans practice fasting as a means of spiritual enlightenment. The greatest modern example of the power of fasting is Mahatma Gandhi, who won India's freedom from the great British Empire in a complete and miraculous nonviolent victory of spiritual leadership.

I cannot overstate the importance of the habit of quiet meditation and prayer for more health of the body, mind and spirit.
"In quietness shall be your strength." – Isaiah 30:15

Fasting brings spiritual rebirth to those who purify their bodies. The light of the world will illuminate within you when you fast. What the eyes are for the outer world, fasts are for the inner. – Mahatma Gandhi

108

My Unforgettable Experience with Gandhi

This is the story of Paul Bragg's meeting with Gandhi told in his own words. *The date I met Mahatma Gandhi was July 27, 1946 in New Delhi, which would become the capital of the new Republic of India a year and a month later. (India's independence became official on August 15, 1947.) At Gandhi's headquarters, I received permission to accompany this amazing man on a 21-day fasting trip eastward through India's villages, where he would walk and talk with the people and help them. At that time, the average Indian earned about 10 cents a day and starvation was a way of life. To show he shared their plight, this compassionate spiritual leader was planning to travel the dusty roads from village to village on foot, without food, only water for 3 weeks.*

Gandhi – A Spiritual Miracle

Gandhi was then 77 years of age and looked frail in appearance. But looks were indeed deceiving! This man was a tower of strength . . . physically, mentally and spiritually. His stamina, endurance, energy and mental abilities were astounding to everyone, including me!

The trek began at sunup. The heat and humidity were the worst I have ever experienced. I have spent time in some of the hottest places in the world, including Death Valley in California, the Sahara Desert and North Africa on an 800-mile bicycle trip in the summer. But never once did Gandhi seem to tire. Never once did he falter in his brisk pace of walking. The only time he sat down was during talks with the villagers. He would speak for 20 minutes, then answer questions for 20 minutes. Then we continued down the hot, dusty road to the next village. Gandhi ate nothing and drank only water flavored with lemon and honey.

Brisk walking is king of exercise! With walking you discover the beauty of nature and it awakens and softens your soul and life!
– Patricia Bragg

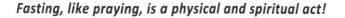

Fasting, like praying, is a physical and spiritual act!

Many who tried to travel with him fell by the wayside, suffering from heat and exhaustion. But Gandhi was inexhaustible! I have been an athlete and hiker all my life, but I have never seen anyone who had the physical stamina and energy that Gandhi had. Each day he walked and talked until sundown before stopping for a rest. During the 21-day fasting walk, I had many talks with Gandhi on the power of fasting. Of all I learned from him, this one statement seems to me the summation:

"All the vitality and energy I have comes to me because my body is purified by fasting." – Gandhi

Walking miles from village to village, he gave people courage and hope that a better life was coming to them! (It has, India won.) His internal strength and beautiful pure soul were so powerful that weak people felt strong after seeing him and hearing his wisdom. He gave his unlimited strength to the discouraged and the sick. He brought a bright light and love where there was darkness. Gandhi told the people that there is truth in the saying that man becomes what he eats.

"Fasting Brings Spiritual Rebirth to All Who Cleanse and Purify Their Bodies."

Gandhi told everyone to fast and purify their bodies and they would find real peace and joy on earth.

"The light of the world will illuminate within you, when you fast and purify yourself." – Gandhi

This trip with the great Gandhi is an experience I will never forget! This physically small man was a spiritual giant. He led millions of people to independence from the mighty British Empire without striking a single physical blow. Yet, with all his power and influence, he was completely without arrogance. Characteristically, on the day of India's independence, Gandhi took no part in the celebrations that went on; instead he spent the day in fasting and prayer in his garden.

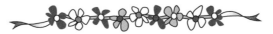

 Often food can cloud what God wants to say to us, so we fast to reveal His wise revelations.

The Grotto Where Jesus Fasted

A story by Paul Bragg in his own words: *On one of my trips to the Holy Land, I was in the area of Jericho. It was near the Mount of Temptation, where Jesus is said to have been tempted by the devil after his fast of 40 days and 40 nights. I decided to climb it. It was a long, easy ascent. From the top, which was still 200 feet below sea level, I looked down upon the hot, barren Jordan Valley. On my descent, halfway down, I came upon a monastery built partly within the rock itself where 10 elderly Greek monks were living in poverty. Following the ancient custom of greeting any stranger as if he might be a wandering Christ, these monks welcomed me with beautiful courtesy. I was taken on a tour of the monastery. It was a fantastic place; parts of it jutted out over deep, brutal chasms while other rooms were carved out of the solid rock. One of these was a grotto which, my guide told me, was "the very spot where Jesus fasted 40 days and 40 nights."*

Fasting Keeps Monks Youthful

The monks told me that they fasted two days every week, and once a year they fasted 40 days and nights in the grotto. They felt that this fasting not only gave them great spiritual enlightenment, but added vigorous, healthy years to their lives. Their youthful appearance bore out their belief. Though far along in calendar years, these men had great flexibility. It required a lot of stamina to keep the monastery in good condition in this rugged, barren wilderness and oven-like heat. All were healthy, lean and muscular, with the glow of health to their skin and bright, keen eyes – none of them wore glasses!

Their spiritual quality showed in the genuine brotherly love which they bestowed on me, a complete stranger. At the end of my visit, one of the monks escorted me to the gate, kissed me on both cheeks and gave me a Greek blessing.

Biblical fasting as with praying and giving are a normal part of our walk with God is taken for granted by the Lord Jesus. Immediately following the Lord's Prayer, He said: "Moreover when ye fast . . . " – Matthew 6

Looking back, as I descended the long, stony trail, I saw him watching. We waved to each other and I carried a warm glow of friendliness in my heart from that barren rocky land. Here again was proof of what I have learned from my own experience – that one of the spiritual benefits of fasting is an empowerment of genuine sense of service, kinship and love for all humanity.

The Fast of 40 Days and 40 Nights

There is a significance to the "40 days and 40 nights" of fasting of the great spiritual leaders and of those who seek the highest spiritual enlightenment. This is the practical limit to which the disciplined body can exist without food before it begins to consume itself. The cleansing process has been completed, and all toxic wastes and excess fat have been "incinerated" – or burned up into energy. When this limit is reached, starvation begins. The body will then have to feed on sound living tissue and this is harmful to body, mind and spirit! The fast should be terminated before this point! A long fast should never be attempted until the body has been trained to fast for short intervals, of up to 10 days, over a period of time.

We don't advise a 40-day fast, it is not for the novice! It's only the experienced faster who learns to distinguish between the early cravings of habitual appetite and the warning pangs of genuine hunger cry for food.

At the beginning of a fast there is a craving for food which arises from the habit of eating at certain intervals. This may last for several days, and then the craving passes. There follows a short period of several days or more when the faster might feel some weakness and require more rest. This may be the most difficult period of the fast.

Jesus fasted 40 days and 40 nights and was filled with the Power of the Holy Spirit. Before Jesus fasted there were no miracles. After His fast God's gifts were in operation in His life. Then Jesus begins His miracle healing ministry.

I humbled my soul with fasting. – Psalm 69:10

Gradually this sense of weakness will disappear, signalling the body has eliminated its worst wastes and toxins. Then comes a feeling of growing strength, with little or no concern for food, and an increasing mental alertness. There is a sense of release and freedom as one ascends to the higher levels of serenity and peace of mind. Spiritual awareness can reach a point of ecstasy!

How long this fasting period lasts depends on the individual. When the process of elimination of all wastes has been completed, the body signals a warning with pangs of genuine hunger. When this happens, whether after 2, 3 or, 4 weeks, the fast must end to preserve all its benefits!

A Sound Mind in a Sound Body

Even the greatest spiritual leaders that the world has known trained themselves by habitual fasting, 1 or 2 days a week, before they undertook longer fasts. Herein lies the difference between genuine healthy fasting and extreme asceticism, which has given fasting a bad name by prolonging it into starvation, which is wrong.

True fasting is healing for the mind, spirit and body. It's truly a natural miracle to achieve "a sound mind in a sound body," or as the Greeks have put it:

"Your body is a temple of the Holy Spirit."

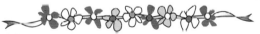

God gave His creatures light, air and water open to the skies;
man locks him in a stifling lair, then wonders why his brother dies.
– Oliver Wendell Holmes

Miracles come with prayer and fasting. – Mark 9:29

Is this not the fast I choose to loosen the bonds of evil,
to undo the heavy burdens, and to let the oppressed
go free and break every yoke? – Isaiah 58:6

The way Jesus sought-after spiritual gifts was to fast.

Stagnation in the body results in premature ageing and also illness.
Fasting promotes cleansing and healing and reversal of ageing.

Paul C. Bragg Found Peace, Relaxation and Joy – and then Crusaded to Share it with the World!

Many people talk about relaxing – just as I used to talk about. But only after years of consistent healthy lifestyle living with fasting and purification did I really learn to completely relax! Each day I'm able to release all tensions from my nerves and muscles and thus renew my vitality and energy through complete relaxation. I sleep better now than I did when I was a child! I find that no matter where I am – no matter what the noise or excitement may be – I can sit or lie down, close my eyes and completely relax. This I want for you also!

I find I'm able to understand other people now when they become upset and emotional. I'm therefore better able to help them calm down. I feel I'm growing – and not only on the physical side! I believe I'm not only building a powerful physical body but, through cleansing and fasting, I'm also advancing mentally and spiritually. I constantly search for light, truth and education along all lines. I find I have a greater interest in everything that is happening in the world. I find I understand people better and in understanding others, I'm able to better understand myself. This way of life opens many doors that lead to a higher life! After all, as we journey through life we should grow and balance our lives physically, mentally, emotionally and spiritually. Many of our worldwide health followers write us about this newly discovered strength in mental and spiritual growth they are experiencing. They rejoice when they have found peace in their mind, soul and total being. **This is the true joy of healthy living!**

I'm a happy man! I have no worries, no fears and no false ambitions! I lead a simple, healthy, happy fulfilled life and give thanks for all my blessings daily! **with love,**
Remember Patricia and I are your health friends for eternity. Paul C. Bragg

---

Dear friend, I wish above all things that thou may prosper and be in health even as the soul prospers. – 3 John 2

Nothing in all creation is so like God as soothing stillness. – Meister Eckhart

Chapter 22

The Science of Eating For Super Health

It is the consensus of opinion among most people that we eat, *"To keep up our strength."* This association of food and strength has been so driven into our subconscious mind that we feel we must eat heavy, rich foods three times a day. *"Something that sticks to the ribs,"* people say. A person who has a big appetite is often falsely thought of as a healthy person. If we know a person who has been sick, and they are encouraged when they're able to sit up and take nourishment, even if in the hospital, that is generally thought of as a healthy action.

During our long study and research into the value of food, we have come to regard nourishment as something more than habitual eating. The body can be fed with anything that is put into the stomach to subdue hunger. Food, however, and nutrition plays an important role in our lives because the body is built from the food we eat. With food we either build strong, disease-free, youthful cells or we build sick cells . . . cells that do not support us as they should. We see a lot of people who are amply-fed, but they are far from well-nourished! They have poor skin and muscle tone and lack health and energy, even though plenty of food is going into their bodies.

115

At one time in our early history, when our food came exclusively from Mother Nature, unprocessed and with no toxic chemicals – we had a natural attraction to the kind of food our body needed. We had a superior sensitivity in our selection of food for life. In other words, there was an inner voice that told us what to eat. We can call it a God-given instinct, that the animals in nature possess. We were, in early times, naturally healthy, beautiful specimens as the early Greeks and Romans were.

Fasting restores a natural, normal appetite when the fast is broken.

Keep Healthy on the Alkaline Diet

Please understand that this program of eating is designed to give you the best nourishment that the food of civilization can offer you. At the same time, the suggested menus that follow are also for cleansing and purification. That is, you must look upon all organic fruits and vegetables not only as protective foods, but foods that are filled with minerals, vitamins, enzymes and valuable nutrients. Foods that are highly alkaline will help keep your alkaline and acid levels balanced.

Many people studying nutrition become confused because there are so many opposing opinions! Some nutritionists advise a high-protein diet. Some promote a low-carbohydrate diet and some endorse a raw fruit, raw vegetable or lacto-vegetarian diet. Each authority says his is the best. We respect every scientist's views in the study of nutrition. We believe that it is impossible to lay down absolute nutritional laws except when it comes to dead, devitalized, demineralized, processed, sprayed and empty-calorie commercial fast foods that are junk foods of our present day modern civilization!

Today we have a selection of over 200 foods. You can build a healthy, delicious, adequate diet around all of them. As you fast and cleanse, you purify your body. And as you cleanse your body, your body itself will guide you naturally to make selections of healthy foods that are right for your body. The main thing is to eliminate the processed foods of modern civilization. It's not so much a question of what you eat as what you shouldn't eat. We have given you the list of foods to avoid (see page 127). There is an old cliche that says, *"A man is either his own doctor at 40 or he is a fool."* We must say here that we believe that any person 30 years of age who is not his own conscientious health captain is very soon going to run into some very serious physical health problems!

The accumulation of toxins in the body accelerates ageing.
The elimination of toxins awakens capacity for renewal.
Toxins must be identified and eliminated from your body.
Fasting is Mother Nature's and God's cleansing miracle!

Activity Draws on Your Vital Force's Energy

Our physical and mental activity draws heavily on our Vital Force. Each of us has different demands. We push ourselves physically because we enjoy physical activity. We enjoy mental activity. We like problems and we enjoy the challenge of solving them. We don't like to live a soft life physically or mentally. We are seekers of spiritual light, comfort, tranquility and serenity. All of this takes our body's Vital Force's energy.

One cannot give simple answers about nutrition. The nutritionist can give you a lot of vital information, but they cannot eat for you or digest for you or eliminate for you! What we eat may not suit your needs, your likes or dislikes. We don't eat as much food as the average person seems to crave and desire.

Every human is unique, as each snowflake is different. We are not trying to persuade you into fast changes. But if you want to feel superior health you must eat a diet of simple, natural healthy foods. We are not going to tell you to become a raw food eater, a strict vegetarian, a lacto-vegetarian or a mixed eater. As you fast and purify, an inner voice, your natural instinct will gradually assert itself. We don't believe that you can quickly jump from a highly refined diet to a natural food diet overnight.

117

Mother Nature doesn't heal in sudden jolts. You ate in a certain pattern for many years, and your digestive and vital organs have adjusted themselves to an unhealthy diet. So move slowly. By body purification through fasting and adhering to the dictates of the *Nine Natural Doctors* (see page 61), you will soon be enjoying the same super health as we do, plus millions of our Bragg followers. In time you will instinctively select natural, healthy foods.

Fasting breaks the addiction to junk food!
Many people are in bondage to food, similar to dealing
with alcohol, drugs, tobacco or any other addictions.
Faithful fasting for only a few days can begin to
help break these addictions.

Work Towards a Balanced, Natural Diet

Building a good nutritional program is like climbing a ladder. There is the first rung – the elimination of all the devitalized, commercial, dead foods of modern life. This means the elimination of all unhealthy beverages – coffee, tea, alcohol, soft drinks and chemicalized waters. It means slowly reducing the amount of animal products you eat – eggs and dairy products. It means adding more raw organic fruits, salads and vegetables to your diet until the total amount of raw food in your diet is between 60% and 70%. As we said earlier, when adding more fruits, salads and vegetables, move slowly!

This period of discarding devitalized foods of civilization and adding more fruits and vegetables is known as the "transition diet." Most people, from childhood until death, live on a diet that is predominantly acidic. Wrong foods produce autointoxication, and this toxic material causes aches, pains, inflammation, and degeneration of the body. So, if you have been living on a diet with mostly heavily cooked foods – such as meats, eggs, refined white breads, spaghetti, chips, pastries, cookies, let us warn you to move slowly and slowly add raw fruits and vegetables. After each weekly fast, you will be able to enjoy and will want more raw fruits, salads, greens and raw veggies, because fasting is purifying your body!

118

Eat Simple, Natural Foods to Stay Healthy

After three months of faithfully fasting one day a week, you will be able to add at least 40% more raw fruits and vegetables to your diet. Remember these raw foods are the purifiers, cleansers and detoxifiers. They dig down into the old pockets of toxic poison and flush them out. This is how you can attain a superior state of radiant health! You are now going to keep internally clean and healthy.

Life cannot be maintained unless life can be taken in. This is best done by making at least 60% of your diet raw and with a plentiful supply of fresh juicy organic fruits along with some lightly cooked vegetables.
– Patricia Bragg

People often ask us, *"Give me the perfect diet."* This is what we cannot do because eating is so personal – we can only suggest that you reread and study the food lists that we have included in this book so you can find foods that appeal to you and benefit your health (see pages 120-122).

Nutrition is like a chain in which all essential items are separate links. If the chain is weak or broken at any point the whole chain fails. If there are 40 items that are essential to the healthy diet, and one of these is missing, nutrition fails just as if half the links were missing. The lack of any item (or several items) can result in ill health. An insufficient amount of any one item is enough to bring distress to the cells and tissues. It is not necessary that every item be furnished at every meal, or every day, because our bodies always carry some reserves.

Here are some healthy foods you can select when building your healthy diet. You can divide your daily nutrition into one, two or three meals. As we mentioned before, we don't eat a heavy breakfast. If you call an Energy Smoothie (page 124) or fresh fruit a breakfast, then that is our breakfast. We are not advising this practice for everyone; some prefer a large breakfast and a small lunch. Everyone's desires are different. We feel that we don't need breakfast and we have explained why (see page 19). Keep a daily journal (page 126) to allow yourself to learn what fuels and feeds your body optimally.

Morning Resolve To Start Your Day

I will this day live a simple, sincere and serene life; repelling promptly every thought of impurity, discontent, anxiety, fear, and discouragement. I will cultivate health, cheerfulness, happiness, charity and the love of brotherhood; exercising economy in expenditure, generosity in giving, carefulness in conversation and diligence in appointed service. I pledge fidelity to every trust and a childlike faith in God. I will be faithful in those habits of prayer, study, work, nutrition, physical exercise, deep breathing and good posture. I shall fast for a 24-hour period each week, eat only healthy foods and get sufficient sleep each night. I will make every effort to improve myself – physically, mentally, emotionally and spiritually every day.

Morning Prayer used by Patricia Bragg & her father, Paul C. Bragg

Fruit – the Most Healthy Food for Man

Here is our fresh fruit list. We regard fruit as the prize food of man. Fresh fruit or sun dried fruit can be used as a meal in itself, or it can be used as a dessert. Make sure that all the fruit you consume is organic.

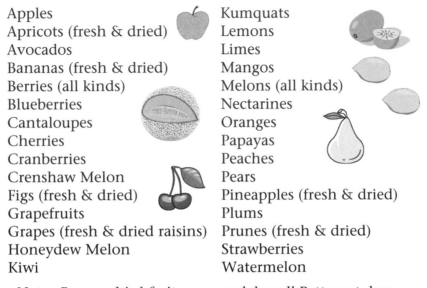

Apples
Apricots (fresh & dried)
Avocados
Bananas (fresh & dried)
Berries (all kinds)
Blueberries
Cantaloupes
Cherries
Cranberries
Crenshaw Melon
Figs (fresh & dried)
Grapefruits
Grapes (fresh & dried raisins)
Honeydew Melon
Kiwi

Kumquats
Lemons
Limes
Mangos
Melons (all kinds)
Nectarines
Oranges
Papayas
Peaches
Pears
Pineapples (fresh & dried)
Plums
Prunes (fresh & dried)
Strawberries
Watermelon

120

Note: Be sure dried fruits are unsulphured! Better yet, buy a dehydrator & enjoy making your own delicious dried organic fruits.

Raw, Unsalted Nut and Seed List

The next list that we will share with you is that of nuts and seeds. They are rich in protein, oils, fiber and micronutrients. You can select any two of the nuts and seeds when you are planning a meal. Enjoy nuts or seeds for your protein. If you have tender gums or unreliable dentures, purchase an electric coffee grinder to make it easier to masticate, assimilate and digest nuts and seeds or eat commercially organically grown nut butter.

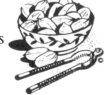

Almonds
Brazil Nuts
Cashew Nuts
Chestnuts
Filberts
Hazelnuts
Hemp Seeds, hulled

Macadamia Nuts
Pecans
Pine Nuts
Pumpkin Seeds
Sesame Seeds
Sunflower Seeds
Walnuts

Organic Vegetables – Purifiers & Protectors

When planning your perfect health meals, select the raw vegetables for your salad from this list. For the largest meal of the day, select one green and one yellow vegetable or you can select any other two vegetables from this list for your cooked vegetables:

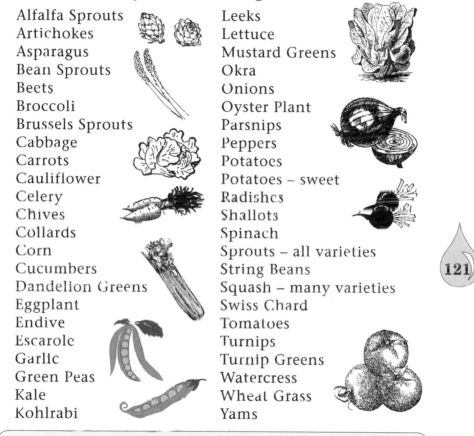

Alfalfa Sprouts
Artichokes
Asparagus
Bean Sprouts
Beets
Broccoli
Brussels Sprouts
Cabbage
Carrots
Cauliflower
Celery
Chives
Collards
Corn
Cucumbers
Dandelion Greens
Eggplant
Endive
Escarole
Garlic
Green Peas
Kale
Kohlrabi

Leeks
Lettuce
Mustard Greens
Okra
Onions
Oyster Plant
Parsnips
Peppers
Potatoes
Potatoes – sweet
Radishes
Shallots
Spinach
Sprouts – all varieties
String Beans
Squash – many varieties
Swiss Chard
Tomatoes
Turnips
Turnip Greens
Watercress
Wheat Grass
Yams

Enjoy Organic Beans and Legumes

Our next list is that of beans and legumes, which are some of man's oldest foods. They are healthy, hearty foods everyone can enjoy. They're rich in vegetable proteins, particularly soybeans (see page 123).

Beans (all kinds)
Garbanzo Beans

Lentils
Lima Beans

Soybeans
Split Peas

Nutrition directly affects growth, development, reproduction, well-being and an individual's physical and mental condition. Health depends upon nutrition more than on any other single factor. – Dr. William H. Sebrell, Jr.

Natural Sweeteners

Here now are some natural sweeteners. Remember they are concentrated sugars and should be used sparingly:

Honey – raw, uncooked   Date Sugar – from dates
100% Maple Syrup   Molasses – unsulphured
Barley Malt   Blackstrap Molasses
Rice Syrup/Malt   Fruit Juices (concentrate)

* Or if you would like to use a zero glycemic, sugar-free sweetener you may use *Stevia herb* (page 84) or Monk Fruit Powder.

Natural Healthy Oils

Next is our list of healthy natural oils. These oils are unsaturated but still use them sparingly. Read the labels: refuse oils that contain chemicals to prevent rancidity. Organic cold-pressed or expeller-pressed oils available at health stores are the best.

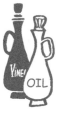

Organic Extra-Virgin Olive Oil   Soy Oil
Organic Macadamia Nut Oil   Corn Oil
Hemp Seed Oil   Sesame Oil
Safflower Oil   Avocado Oil
Flaxseed Oil   Walnut Oil
Sunflower Oil   Almond Oil

122

Natural Organic Whole Grains, Flours & Cereals

These 100% whole grains are best for health. Cereals should not be eaten more than three times a week unless you do physical heavy labor or heavy sports training, because they are very acidic. On your cereal you may use any of the natural sweetening agents and rice, almond or oat milks.

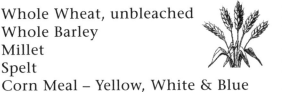

Whole Wheat, unbleached   Rye
Whole Barley   Flax
Millet   Quinoa
Spelt   Kamut
Corn Meal – Yellow, White & Blue   Amaranth
Oats – steel cut oats (a Bragg favorite) Buckwheat
Brown Rice – organic & unrefined   Bulgur
Organic Rice – long & short grain, Basmati & Wild Rice

Plant-Based Protein Chart

BEANS & LEGUMES

(1 cup cooked)	PROTEIN IN GRAMS
Soybeans	29
Lentils	18
Adzuki Beans	17
Cannellini	17
Navy Beans	16
Split Peas	16
Black Beans	15
Garbanzos (chick peas)	15
Kidney Beans	15
Great Northern Beans	15
Lima Beans	15
Black-eyed Peas	14
Pinto Beans	14
Mung Beans	14
Tofu (3 oz.)	7 to 12
Green Peas (whole)	9

RAW NUTS & SEEDS

(¼ cup or 4 Tbsps)	PROTEIN IN GRAMS
Chia Seeds	12
Macadamia Nuts	11
Flax Seeds	8
Sunflower Seeds	8
Almonds	7
Pumpkin Seeds	7
Sesame Seeds	7
Walnuts	5
Brazil Nuts	5
Hazelnuts	5
Pine Nuts	4
Cashews	4

NUT BUTTERS

(2 Tbsps)	PROTEIN IN GRAMS
Peanut Butter	7 to 9
Almond Butter	5 to 8
Cashew Butter	4 to 5
Sesame - Tahini	6

VEGETABLES

(1 Serving or 1 cup)	PROTEIN IN GRAMS
Spirulina	8.6
Corn (1 cob)	5
Potato (with skin)	5
Mushrooms, Oyster	5
Artichoke (1 medium)	4
Collard Greens	4
Broccoli	4
Brussel Sprouts	4
Mushrooms, Shitake	3.5
Swiss Chard	3
Kale	2.5
Asparagus (5 spears)	2
String Beans	2
Beets	2
Peas	2
Sweet Potato	3
Summer Squash	2
Cabbage	2
Carrot	2
Cauliflower	2
Squash	2
Celery	1
Spinach	1
Bell Peppers	1
Cucumber	1
Eggplant	1
Leeks	1
Lettuce	1
Tomato (1 medium)	1
Radish	1
Turnips	1

DAIRY & NUT MILKS

(1 cup)	PROTEIN IN GRAMS
Soy Milk	6 to 9
Almond Milk	1 to 2
Rice Milk	1
Eggs (1) *(free-range)*	6

FRUITS

(1 Serving or 1 cup)	PROTEIN IN GRAMS
Avocado (1 medium)	4
Banana (1)	1 to 2
Blackberries (1 cup)	2
Pomegranate (1)	1.5
Blueberries (1 cup)	1
Cantaloupe (1 cup)	1
Cherries (1 cup)	1
Grapes (1 cup)	1
Honeydew (1 cup)	1
Kiwi (1 large)	1
Lemon (1)	1
Mango (1)	1
Nectarine (1)	1
Orange (1)	1
Peach (1)	1
Pear (1)	1
Pineapple (1 cup)	1
Plum (1)	1
Raspberries (1 cup)	1
Strawberries (1 cup)	1
Watermelon (1 cup)	1

123

GRAINS & RICE

(1 cup cooked)	PROTEIN IN GRAMS
Triticale	25
Millet	8.4
Amaranth	7
Oat Bran	7
Wild Rice	7
Couscous (whole wheat)	6
Bulgar Wheat	6
Buckwheat	6
Teff	6
Oat Groats	6
Barley	5
Quinoa	5
Brown Rice	5
Spelt	5

This chart displays protein content of common vegetarian foods.

Note that in order to determine amount of protein that is optimal for your body, use the following formula that is based on a vegan diet: *RDA recommends that we take in 0.36 grams of protein per pound that we weigh* (100 lbs. x 0.36 = 36 grams).

Data from webs: *TheHolyKale.com • VegParadise.com • vrg.org (Vegetarian Resource Group).*

HEALTHY BEVERAGES
Fresh Juices, Herb Teas & Energy Drinks

These freshly squeezed organic vegetable and fruit juices are important to *The Bragg Healthy Lifestyle*. It's not wise to drink beverages with your main meals, as it dilutes the digestive juices. But it's great during the day to have a glass of freshly squeezed orange juice, grapefruit juice, vegetable juice, raw, organic apple cider vinegar drink (see below), or herbal tea – these are all ideal pick-me-up beverages.

Apple Cider Vinegar Drink – Mix 1-2 tsps. raw, organic apple cider vinegar (with the 'Mother' enzyme) and (optional) to taste raw honey or pure maple syrup *(if diabetic, to sweeten use 2 stevia drops)* in 8 oz. of distilled or purified water. Take glass upon arising, hour before lunch and dinner.

Delicious Hot or Cold Cider Drink – Add 2-3 cinnamon sticks and 4 cloves to water and boil. Steep 20 minutes or more. Before serving add raw organic apple cider vinegar and sweetener to taste.

Bragg's Favorite Juice Drink – This drink consists of all raw vegetables *(remember organic is best)* which we prepare in our juicer / blender: carrots, celery, cucumber, beets, cabbage, tomatoes, watercress, kale, parsley, or any vegetable combination you prefer. The great purifier, garlic we enjoy, but it's optional.

Bragg's Favorite Healthy Energy Smoothie – After morning stretch and exercises we often enjoy the drink below instead of fruit. It's a delicious and powerfully nutritious meal anytime: lunch, dinner or in a thermos at work, school, sports, the gym and during sports or hikes. You can freeze for popsicles too.

Bragg's Favorite Healthy Energy Smoothie

(124)

Prepare the following in a blender, add frozen juice cubes if desired colder; Choice of: freshly squeezed orange or grapefruit juice; carrot and greens juice; unsweetened pineapple juice; or 1 1/2 - 2 cups purified or distilled water with:

2 tsps spirulina or green powder	1-2 bananas or fresh fruit
1/3 tsp nutritional yeast	1-2 tsps almond or nut butter
2 dates or prunes-pitted	1 tsp flaxseed oil or grind seeds
1 tsp protein powder (optional)	1 tsp raw honey (optional)

Optional: 4-6 apricots (sun-dried,) soak in jar overnight in purified water or unsweetened pineapple juice. We soak enough to last for several days. Keep refrigerated. In summer you can add organic fresh fruit: peaches, papaya, blueberries, strawberries, all berries, apricots, etc. instead of banana. In winter, add apples, kiwi, oranges, tangelos, persimmons or pears, and if fresh is unavailable, try sugar-free, frozen organic fruits. Serves 1 to 2.

Patricia's Delicious Health Popcorn

Use freshly popped organic popcorn (use air popper). Drizzle organic olive oil, melted coconut oil or salt-free butter over popcorn. Sprinkle with good quality nutritional yeast for amazing flavor. For a variety try a pinch of cayenne pepper, mustard powder or fresh crushed garlic to oil mixture. Serve instead of breads!

Seek and choose whole foods, organic fruits, vegetables and organic whole grain cereals, breads, etc. rather than commercial, canned, refined white flour, sugar products and other highly processed goods in the center aisles.

Lentil & Brown Rice Casserole, Burgers or Soup
Paul Bragg and Jack LaLanne's Favorite Recipe

16 oz pkg organic lentils, uncooked
1 cup brown organic rice, uncooked
5 cups, distilled / purified water
4-6 carrots, chop ¹/₂" rounds
3 celery stalks, chop

4 garlic cloves, chop
2 onions, chop
2 tsps organic coconut aminos
1 tsp salt-free all-purpose seasoning
2 tsps organic extra-virgin olive oil

1 cup diced fresh or canned tomatoes (salt-free)

Wash and drain lentils and rice. Place grains in large stainless steel pot. Add water, bring to boil, reduce heat and simmer 30 minutes. Now add vegetables and seasonings and cook on low heat until tender. Last five minutes add fresh or canned (salt-free) tomatoes. For delicious garnish, add minced parsley. **For Burgers mash. For Soup, add more water in cooking grains.** Serves 4 to 6.

Raw Organic Vegetable Health Salad

2 stalks celery, chop
1 bell pepper & seeds, dice
¹/₂ cucumber, slice
2 carrots, grate
1 raw beet, grate
1 cup green cabbage, chop

¹/₂ cup red cabbage, chop
¹/₂ cup alfalfa, mung or sunflower sprouts
2 spring onions & green tops, chop
1 turnip, grate
1 avocado (ripe)
3 tomatoes, medium size

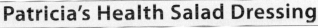

For variety add organic raw zucchini, peas, mushrooms, broccoli, cauliflower, (try black olives and pasta). Chop, slice or grate vegetables fine to medium for variety in size. Mix vegetables & serve on bed of lettuce, spinach, chopped kale or cabbage. Dice avocado and tomato and serve on side as a dressing. Serve choice of fresh squeezed lemon, orange or dressing separately. Chill salad plates before serving. **It's best to always eat salad first before hot dishes.** Serves 3 to 5.

125

Patricia's Health Salad Dressing

¹/₂ cup raw organic apple cider vinegar
1-2 tsps organic raw honey

¹/₂ tsp organic coconut aminos
1-2 cloves garlic, minced

¹/₃ cup organic extra-virgin olive oil, or blend with safflower, soy, sesame or flax oil
1 Tbsp fresh herbs, minced (to taste)

Blend ingredients in blender or jar. Refrigerate in covered jar.

For delicious Herbal Vinegar: In quart jar add ¹/₃ cup tightly packed, crushed fresh sweet basil, tarragon, dill, oregano, or any fresh herbs desired, combined or singly (if dried herbs, use 1-2 tsps herbs). Now cover to top with raw, organic apple cider vinegar and store two weeks in warm place, and then strain and refrigerate.

Honey – Chia or Celery Seed Vinaigrette

¹/₄ tsp dry mustard
¹/₄ tsp organic coconut aminos
¹/₄ tsp paprika or to taste
1-2 Tbsps honey

1 cup organic apple cider vinegar
¹/₂ cup organic extra-virgin olive oil
¹/₂ small onion, minced
¹/₃ tsp chia or celery seed (or vary to taste)

Blend ingredients in blender or jar. Refrigerate in covered jar.

Studies show both beta carotene and vitamin C, abundantly found in fruits and vegetables, play vital roles in preventing heart disease and cancers.

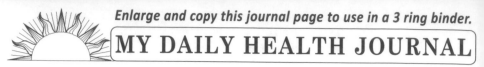

MY DAILY HEALTH JOURNAL

Today is:____/____/____

> *I have said my morning resolve and am ready to practice faithfully The Bragg Healthy Lifestyle today and every day.*

Yesterday I went to bed at: Today I arose at: Weight:

Today I practiced the No-Heavy Breakfast or No-Breakfast Plan: ☐ yes ☐ no

• For Breakfast I drank: Time:

  For Breakfast I ate:
                                                                  Time:
  Supplements:

• For Lunch I ate: Time:

  Supplements:

• For Dinner I ate: Time:

  Supplements:

• ____ Glasses of Water I Drank during the Day, including ACV Drinks

  List Snacks – Kind and When:

_____

• I took part in these physical activities (walking, gym, etc.) today:

_____

Grade each on scale of 1 to 10 (desired optimum health is 10).

• I rate my day for the following categories:

Previous Night's Sleep:	Stress/Anxiety:
Energy Level:	Elimination:
Physical Activity, Exercise:	Health:
Peacefulness:	Accomplishments:
Happiness:	Self-Esteem:

_____

• General Comments, Reactions and any To-Do List:

Chapter 23

The Bragg Healthy Lifestyle

For optimal health with *The Bragg Healthy Lifestyle* we suggest you avoid these processed, refined harmful foods. Once you realize the harm caused to your body by unhealthy refined, chemicalized foods, you will want to eliminate these.

Avoid These Processed, Refined, Harmful Foods:

- **Refined sugar / artificial sweeteners** (toxic aspartame) or their products such as jams, jellies, preserves, marmalades, yogurts, ice cream, sherbets, Jello, cake, candy, cookies, all chewing gum, colas and diet drinks, pies, pastries, and all sugared fruit juices and fruits canned in sugar syrup. (Health Stores have delicious healthy replacements!)

- **White flour products** such as white bread, enriched flours, dumplings, biscuits, buns, gravy, pasta, pancakes, waffles, soda crackers, pizza, ravioli, pies, pastries, cakes, cookies, and ready-mix bakery products.

- **Salted foods:** pretzels, corn chips, potato chips, crackers and nuts.

- **Refined white rice** and pearl barley. ● **Fried fast foods.** ● **Indian ghee.**

- **Refined dry processed cereals** that are sugared, such as cornflakes, etc.

- **Foods that contain Olestra**, palm and cottonseed oil.

- **Peanuts and peanut butter** that contain hydrogenated, hardened oils.

- **Margarine, Saturated fats and hydrogenated oils.**

- **Coffee, soft drinks, teas, alcohol, sugared juices** – even it decaffeinated.

- **Fresh pork / products.** ● **Fried, fatty, greasy meats.** ● **Irradiated GMO foods.**

- **Smoked meats**, such as ham, bacon, sausage and all smoked fish.

- **Luncheon meats**, hot dogs, salami, bologna, corned beef, pastrami.

- **Dried fruits** containing sulphur dioxide – a toxic preservative.

- **Chickens, turkeys and meats injected with hormones** or fed with commercial feed containing any drugs or toxins.

- **Canned soups** – read labels for sugar, salt, starch, flour and preservatives.

- **Foods containing preservatives, additives**, benzoate of soda, salt, sugar, cream of tartar, drugs, irradiated and genetically modified foods.

- **All commercial vinegars:** pasteurized, filtered, distilled, white, malt and synthetic vinegars are dead vinegars! (We use only organic raw, unfiltered apple cider vinegar with "Mother Enzyme" as used in olden times.)

Please follow *The Bragg Healthy Lifestyle* to provide basic, healthy nourishment to maintain your precious health.

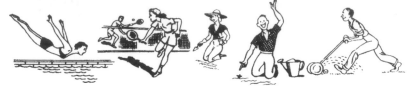

Live The Bragg Healthy Lifestyle
To Enjoy a Lifetime of Super Health!

In a broad sense, *"The Bragg Healthy Lifestyle for the Total Person"* is a combination of physical, mental, emotional, social and spiritual components. The ability of the individual to function effectively in their environment depends on how smoothly these components function as a whole. Of all the qualities that comprise an integrated personality, a totally healthy, fit body is one of the most desirable . . . so start today on your goals for more health, happiness and peace in your life!

A person is said to be totally physically fit if they function as a total personality with efficiency and without pain or discomfort. This is to have a painless, tireless, and ageless body. You possess sufficient muscular strength and endurance to maintain a healthy posture. You can successfully carry on the duties imposed by life and the environment, and meet any emergencies satisfactorily and have enough energy for recreation and social obligations after the "work day" has ended. You possess the body power and Vital Force to recover rapidly from fatigue, and the stress of daily living without the aid of stimulants, drugs or alcohol. You can enjoy recharging sleep at night and awaken fit and alert.

Keeping the body totally healthy and fit is not a job for the uninformed or careless person. It requires an understanding of the body and of a healthy lifestyle and then following that lifestyle for a long, happy life! The purpose of "The Bragg Healthy Lifestyle" is to wake up the possibilities, a rebirth within you, a rejuvenation of your body, mind and spirit for a total balanced body health. It's within your reach, so start today! Daily our hearts and prayers go out to touch your heart and soul with nourishing, caring love for your total health!
With love. your health friends.

Patricia and *Paul C. Bragg*

Ten Tips for Good Health

- *Respect and protect your body as the highest manifestation of your life.*

- *Abstain from unnatural, devitalized foods and stimulating beverages.*

- *Nourish your body with only natural unprocessed, live foods.*

- *Extend your years in health for loving, sharing and charitable service.*

- *Regenerate your body by the right balance of activity and rest.*

- *Purify your cells, tissue and blood with healthy organic foods, and with pure water, clean air and gentle sunshine.*

- *Abstain from all food when out of sorts in mind or body.*

- *Keep thoughts, words and emotions pure, calm, loving and uplifting.*

- *Increase your knowledge of Mother Nature's Laws, follow them, and enjoy the fruits of your life's labor.*

- *Lift up yourself, friends and family by loyal obedience to Mother Nature's and God's Healthy, Natural Laws of Living.*

129

Bragg Healthy Lifestyle Plan

- *Read, plan, plot, and follow through for supreme health and longevity.*

- *Underline, highlight or dog-ear pages as you read important passages.*

- *Organizing your lifestyle helps you identify what's important in your life.*

- *Be faithful to your health goals daily for a healthy, long, fulfilled life.*

- *Where space allows we have included "words of wisdom" from great minds to motivate and inspire you. Please share your favorite sayings with us.*

- *Write us about your successes following The Bragg Healthy Lifestyle.*

Open your eyes so you may behold wondrous things out of Thy law. – Psalm 119:18

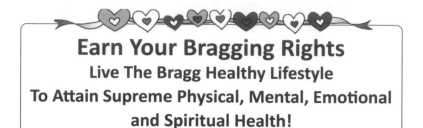

With your new awareness, understanding and sincere commitment of how to live *The Bragg Healthy Lifestyle* – you can now live a longer, healthier life to 120 years! *(Gen. 6:3)*

God bless you and your family and may He give you the strength, the courage and the patience to win your battle to re-enter the Healthy Garden of Eden while you are still living here on Earth with more years to enjoy it all!

With Blessings of Health, Peace, Joy and Love,

Patricia and *Paul C. Bragg*

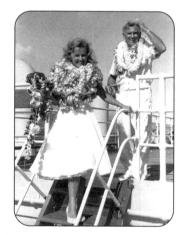

Health Crusaders Paul C. Bragg and daughter Patricia traveled the world spreading health, inspiring millions to renew and revitalize their health.

The Bragg books are written to inspire and guide you to health, fitness and longevity. Remember, the book you don't read won't help. So please reread Bragg Books and live The Bragg Healthy Lifestyle to enjoy a healthy fulfilled life!

I never suspected that I would have to learn how to live – that there were specific disciplines and ways of seeing the world that I had to master before I could awaken to a simple, healthy, happy, uncomplicated life.– Dan Millman, author "The Way of the Peaceful Warrior" • peacefulwarrior.com A Bragg fan and admirer since his Stanford University coaching days.

A truly good book teaches me better than to just read it, I must soon lay it down and commence living in its wisdom. What I began by reading, I must finish by acting! – Henry David Thoreau

Healthy Alternative Therapies
and Massage Techniques

(Try Them – They Are Working Miracles!)

We suggest you explore these wonderful natural methods of healing your body. Finally over 600 Medical Schools in the United States are teaching *Healthy Alternative Therapies*. Please check their websites. Now seek and choose the best healing techniques for you:

ACUPUNCTURE / ACUPRESSURE: Acupuncture directs and rechannels body energy by inserting hair-thin needles (use only disposable needles) at specific points on the body. It's used for pain, backaches, migraines and general health and body dysfunctions. Used in Asia for centuries, acupuncture is safe, virtually painless and has no side effects! Acupressure is based on the same principles and uses finger pressure and massage rather than needles. Check web: *AcupunctureToday.com*

CHIROPRACTIC: was founded in Davenport, Iowa in 1885 by Daniel David Palmer. There are now many schools in the U.S., and graduates are joining Health Practitioners in all nations of the world to share healing techniques. Chiropractic is popular and the largest U.S. healing profession benefitting literally millions! Treatment involves soft tissue, spinal and body adjustment to free your nervous system of any interferences with normal body functions. Its concern is the functional integrity of the musculoskeletal system. In addition to manual methods, chiropractors use physical therapy modalities, exercise, health and nutritional guidance. Web: *ChiroWeb.com*

ALEXANDER TECHNIQUE: helps end improper use of neuromuscular system, helps bring body posture into balance. Eliminates psycho-physical interferences, helps release long-held tension, and aids in re-establishing muscle tone. For more info see web: *AlexanderTechnique.com*

FELDENKRAIS METHOD: Dr. Moshe Feldenkrais founded this in the late 1940s. This Method leads to improved posture and helps create ease and more efficiency of body movement. This Method is a great stress removal. Web: *Feldenkrais.com*

131

Time waits for no one, treasure and protect every moment you have!

HOMEOPATHY: In 1796, Dr. Samuel Hahnemann, a German physician, developed homeopathy. Patients are treated with "micro" doses of remedies found in nature to trigger the body's own defenses. This homeopathic principle is a safe and nontoxic remedy and is the #1 alternative therapy in Europe and Britain because it is inexpensive, seldom has any side effects, and usually brings fast results. Web: *HomeopathyCenter.org*

NATUROPATHY: Brought to America by Dr. Benedict Lust, M.D., this treatment uses diet, herbs, homeopathy, fasting, exercise, hydrotherapy, manipulation and sunlight. Practitioners work with your body to restore health naturally. They reject surgery and drugs except as a last resort. Web: *www.Naturopathic.org*

OSTEOPATHY: The first School of Osteopathy was founded in 1892 by Dr. Andrew Taylor Still, M.D. There are now 30 U.S. colleges. Treatment involves soft tissue, spinal and body adjustments that free the nervous system from interferences that can cause illness. Healing by adjustment also includes good nutrition, physical therapies, proper breathing and good posture. Dr. Still's premise: if the body structure is altered or abnormal, then proper body function is altered and can cause pain and illness. Web: *www.AcademyofOsteopathy.org*

132

REFLEXOLOGY / ZONE THERAPY: Founded by Eunice Ingham, author of *Stories The Feet Can Tell*, inspired by a Bragg Health Crusade when she was 17. Reflexology helps the body and organs by removing crystalline deposits from reflex areas (nerve endings) of feet and hands through deep pressure massage. Primitive reflexology originated in China and Egypt and Native American Indians and Kenyans self-practiced it for centuries. Reflexology activates your body's flow of healing and energy by dislodging deposits. Visit Eunice Ingham and nephew Dwight Byer's website: *www.Reflexology-usa.net*

SKIN BRUSHING: daily is wonderful for circulation, toning, cleansing and healing. Use a dry vegetable brush (never nylon) and brush lightly. Helps purify lymph so it's able to detoxify your blood and tissues. Removes old skin cells, uric acid crystals and toxic wastes that come up through skin's pores. Use loofah sponge for variety in shower or tub.

Skin is often called your third kidney because it eliminates toxins from body.

REIKI: A Japanese form of massage that means "Universal Life Energy." Reiki Massage helps the body to detoxify, then re-balance and heal itself. Discovered in the ancient Sutra manuscripts by Dr. Mikao Usui in Japan 1922. Web: *Reiki.org*

ROLFING: Developed by Ida Rolf in the 1930's in the U.S. Rolfing is also called structural processing and postural release, or structural dynamics. It is based on the concept that distortions (accidents, injuries, falls, etc.) and the effects of gravity on the body cause upsets and long-term stress in the body. Rolfing helps to achieve balance and improved body posture. Methods involve the use of stretching, with gentle deep tissue massage and relaxation techniques to loosen old injuries, break bad movement and posture patterns. Web: *Rolf.org*

TRAGERING: Founded by Dr. Milton Trager M.D., who was inspired at age 18 by Paul Bragg to become a doctor. It is a mind-body learning method that involves gentle shaking and rocking, allowing the body to let go, releasing tensions and lengthening the muscles for more body peace and health. Tragering can do miracle healing where needed in the body frame, muscles and the entire body. Web: *Trager.com*

133

WATER THERAPY: Soothing detox shower: apply olive oil to skin, alternate hot and cold water, every 2-3 minutes. Massage body while under hot, filtered spray. Garden hose massage is great in summer or anytime. Hot detox soak bath (diabetics use warm water) 20 minutes with cup of Epsom salts or apple cider vinegar. This soak helps pull out the toxins by creating an artificial fever cleanse.

COLON HYDROTHERAPY: is a safe and effective practice for supporting detoxification, and improving health and vitality. Contact I-ACT (Int'l Association Colon Hydrotherapy) for a certified colon Hydro-Therapist in your area. Web: *i-act.org*

MASSAGE & AROMATHERAPY: works two ways: the essence (aroma) relaxes, as does healing massages. Essential oils are extracted from flowers, leaves, roots, seeds and barks. These are usually massaged into skin, inhaled or used in a bath to help the body relax, soothe and heal. The oils, used for centuries to treat numerous ailments, are revitalizing and energizing for the body and mind. Web: *www.Aromatherapy.com*

Dad and I want you to enjoy a fulfilled, healthy, long life.
– Patricia Bragg, Pioneer Health Crusader

MASSAGE – SELF: Paul C. Bragg often said, *"You can be your own best massage therapist, even if you have only one good hand."* Near-miraculous health improvements have been achieved by victims of accidents or strokes in bringing life back to afflicted parts of their own bodies by self-massage and with vibrators. Treatments can be day or night, almost continual. Self-massage also helps achieve relaxation at day's end. Families and friends can learn and exchange massages; it's a wonderful sharing experience. Remember, babies love and thrive with daily massages, start from birth. Family pets also love soothing, healing touch of massages. Web: *RD.com/health/wellness/learn-the-art-of-self-massage*

MASSAGE – SHIATSU: Japanese massage form applies pressure from fingers, hands, elbows and even knees along the same points as acupuncture. Shiatsu originated in Japan and is based on traditional Chinese medicine, and has been widely practiced around the world since 1970s. Shiatsu has been used in Asia for centuries to relieve pain, common ills, muscle stress and to aid lymphatic circulation. See web: *centerpointmn.com/the-benefits-of-shiatsu-massage*

134

MASSAGE – SWEDISH: One of the oldest and the most popular and widely used massage techniques. This deep body massage soothes and promotes healthy circulation and is a great way to loosen and relax tight muscles before and after exercise. See web: *www.MassageDen.com/swedish-massage.shtml*

MASSAGE – SPORTS: An important health support system for professional and amateur athletes. Sports massage improves circulation and mobility to injured tissue, enables athletes to recover more rapidly from myofascial injury, reduces muscle soreness and chronic strain patterns. Soft tissues are freed of trigger points and adhesions, thus contributing to improvement of peak neuromuscular functioning and athletic performance.

Author's Comment: We have personally sampled many of these Alternative Therapies. It's estimated that America's health care costs are over $3 trillion. It's more important than ever to be responsible for our own health! This includes seeking dedicated holistic health practitioners to keep us well by inspiring us to practice prevention! These Alternative Healing Therapies are getting results: aromatherapy, Ayurvedic, biofeedback, guided imagery, herbs, hyperbaric oxygen, music, meditation, magnets, saunas, tai chi, Qi gong, Pilates, rebounding, lymphatic drainage therapy, and yoga. Explore them and be open to improving your earthly temple for a healthy, happier, longer life.

Seek and find the best for your body, mind and soul. – Patricia Bragg

BRAGG PHOTO GALLERY

PATRICIA & PAUL C. BRAGG, N.D., Ph.D.
Dynamic Daughter & Father are World Health Crusaders

BRAGG PRODUCTS
HEALTH IS HERE

During the past century, Bragg Live Food Products developed and pioneered the very first line of Health Foods, from vitamins and minerals to organic nuts, seeds, and sun-dried fruits. This included over 365 health products, – *"one for each day of the year!"* says daughter Patricia Bragg.

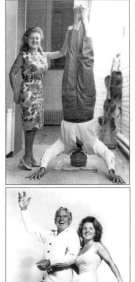

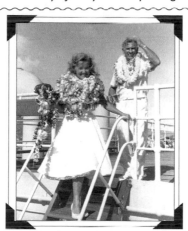

"Thanks for The Bragg Healthy Lifestyle that you shared with me and you are sharing with millions of others worldwide."
– John Gray, Ph.D., author

Picture from
People Magazine August, 1975.

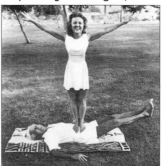

Patricia and father, Paul on world trip in 1950's, during stop in Tahiti.

"You have recharged me with joy, hope, love and encouragement, which poured from your words. I am now fasting and using ACV. You have certainly improved my life!"
– Marie Furia, New Jersey

Patricia Bragg stands on her father's stomach. Paul's stomach muscles are so strong he can lift Patricia up and down!

135

Paul C. BRAGG, N.D., Ph.D.
HEALTH CRUSADER
Life Extension Specialist and Originator of Health Food Stores

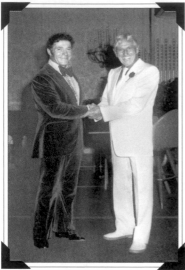

I have experienced a beautiful, remarkable, spiritual and physical awakening since reading Bragg Health Books. I'll never be the same again.
– Sandy Tuttle, Ohio

With every new day comes new strength and new thoughts.
– Eleanor Roosevelt

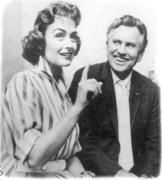

Actress Donna Reed saying "Health First" with Paul C. Bragg.

Dr. Paul C. Bragg (right) Creator Health Food Stores, Pioneer Life Extension Specialist, with his prize student Jack LaLanne. Paul started him on the royal road to health over 85 years ago!

Paul C. Bragg spent much of his time at the Hollywood Studios meeting with top Stars and motion picture industry executives, giving health lectures and private consultations. Dr. Paul C. Bragg was Hollywood's first highly respected, health, fitness and nutrition advisor to the Stars.

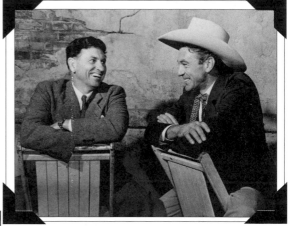

Paul C. Bragg with Gary Cooper, famous American film actor, best known for his many Western films.

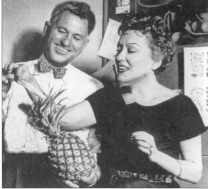

Paul C. Bragg with the famous Hollywood Actress Gloria Swanson, who was leading star in 20s, 30s and 40s. Gloria became a Bragg Health Devotee at 18 and she often would Health Crusade with Bragg during the 1950s.

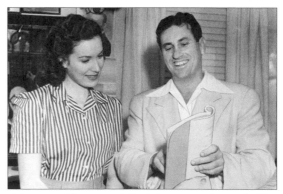

Maureen O'Hara and Paul C. Bragg. This Irish film actress and singer was best noted for playing in "Miracle on 34th Street" and "The Quiet Man."

PAUL C. BRAGG, N.D., Ph.D.
STAYING HEALTHY & FIT

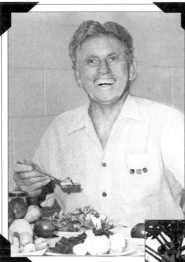

I'd like to thank you for teaching me how to take control of my health! I lost 55 pounds and I feel "great!" Bragg books have showed me vitality, happiness and being close to Mother Nature. You both are real "Crusaders for Health for the World." Thanks!
– Leonard Amato

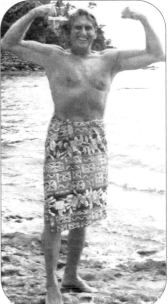

Dr. Paul C. Bragg and daughter Patricia were my early guiding inspiration to my health career.
Jeffery Bland, Ph.D.,
Famous Food Scientist

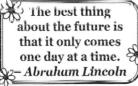
The best thing about the future is that it only comes one day at a time.
– Abraham Lincoln

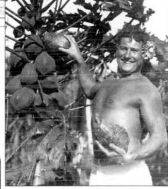

Paul C. Bragg in Tahiti 1920's gathering tropical papaya fruit.

Paul C. Bragg owes his powerful body and superb health to living exclusively on live, vital, healthy, organic rich foods.

Dear Friends – you cannot know how greatly you have impacted my life and some of my friends! We love your Bragg Health Books, teachings and products and are now living healthier, happier lives. Thanks!
– Winnie Brown, Arizona

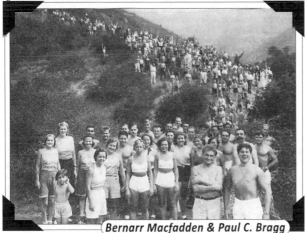

Bernarr Macfadden & Paul C. Bragg

A thousand happy Bragg Health Students enjoy hiking, exercise and fresh air on the trail to Mount Hollywood (above Griffith Observatory) in beautiful California, summer of 1932.

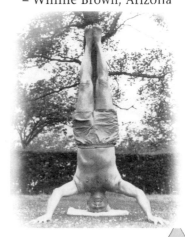

Paul C. Bragg exercising Regent's Park, London.

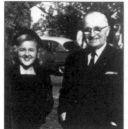

Patricia with 33rd President Harry S. Truman at his home in Independence, Missouri.

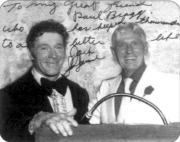

Paul C. Bragg, Creator of Health Food Stores, with his prize student Jack LaLanne, who thanks Bragg for saving his life at 15.

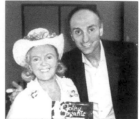

Patrica Bragg with Dr. Jeffrey Smith. He is leader in getting GMO's out of US foods. See GMO video by Jeffrey Smith and narrated by Lisa Oz (Dr. Oz's wife) on web: *GeneticRouletteMovie.com*

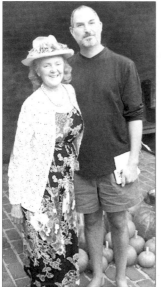

Patricia visiting with Steve Jobs at his home in Palo Alto during the Thanksgiving Holidays.

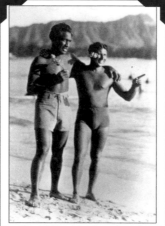

Paul in 1920 with his swimming & surfing friend, Duke Kahanamoku, Waikiki Beach, Diamond Head.

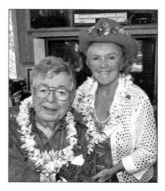

Dr. Earl Bakken with Patricia. He's famous for inventing the first Transistor Pacemaker. His firm Medtronic, developed it and a Resuscitator for fixing ailing hearts that have and are saving thousands of lives. Dr. Bakken lived In Hawaii.

"I've been reading Bragg Books since high school. I'm thankful for the Bragg Healthy Lifestyle and admire their Health Crusading for a healthier, happier world."
– Steve Jobs, Creator –
Apple Computer

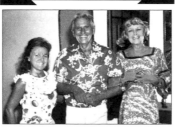

Patricia, Paul C. Bragg and Mrs. Duke (Nadine) Kahanamoku. (Nadine is Patricia's Godmother).

"I cannot remember a time when the Golden Rule was not my motto and precept, the torch that guided my footsteps."* – J.C. Penney

*The Golden Rule: Do unto others as you would have them do unto you.

J.C. Penney & Patricia → exercising. They walked often in Palm Springs when he and his wife visited in the winter to enjoy the warm desert sunshine.

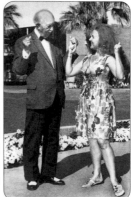

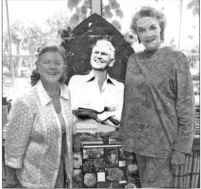

Patricia with friend Actress Jane Russell. Famous Hollywood Star of 40s to 60s.

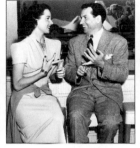

Jane Wyatt learning about health with Paul C. Bragg.

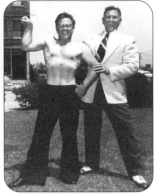

Mickey Rooney with Paul. Rooney was an American film actor and entertainer. He won multiple awards and had one of the longest careers of any actor to age 93!

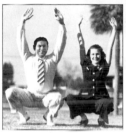

Paul C. Bragg exercising with Actress Helen Parrish.

"Thank you Paul & Patricia Bragg for my simple, easy-to follow Healthy Lifestyle. You make my days healthy!" – Clint Eastwood, Academy Award Winning Film Producer, Director, Actor and Bragg follower for over 65 years.

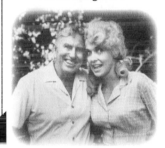

Paul C. Bragg and Donna Douglas, one of Hollywood's most beautiful and talented health advocates. She played the part of "Elly May" in the *Beverly Hillbillies*, which became one of the longest-running series in television history and was the #1 show in America in its first 2 years.

Life is a Miracle
Minute by Minute
Year by Year!

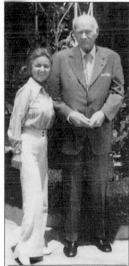

Patricia with Conrad Hilton

← Hotel founder, Conrad Hilton with Patricia Bragg, his Healthy Lifestyle Teacher. *"I wouldn't be alive today if it wasn't for the Braggs and their Bragg Healthy Lifestyle!"* – Conrad Hilton

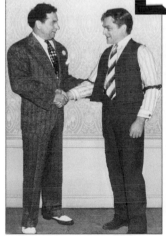

Paul with James Cagney, American film actor. He won major awards for wide variety of roles. The American Film Institute ranked Cagney 8th among the Greatest Male Hollywood Stars of All Time.

"Thank you for your website. What a wealth of info to learn about how to live and eat healthy. Many Blessings!" – Michel & Mary, California

PAUL C. BRAGG, N.D., Ph.D.
PROMOTES HEALTH & FITNESS!

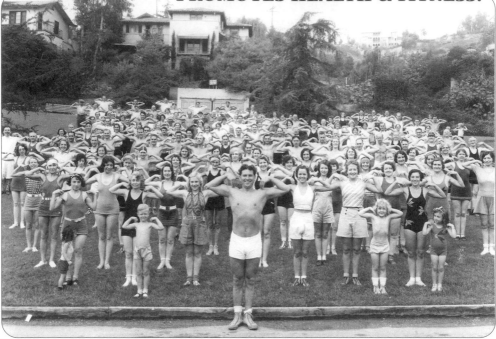

Paul C. Bragg leading an exercise class in Griffith Park, Hollywood, CA – circa 1920s.

Bragg Healthy Lifestyle works Miracles! – Jack LaLanne

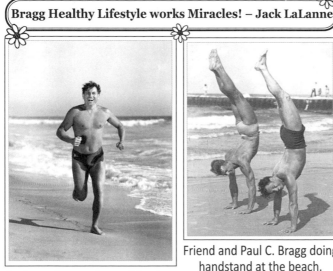

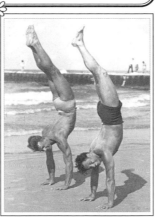

Friend and Paul C. Bragg doing handstand at the beach.

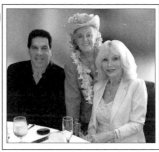

Patricia with Lou and wife Carla at Elaine LaLanne's 90th Birthday Party.

Paul running on Coney Island, New York, where he was a member of the Coney Island Polar Bear Club, known for Cold Water Swimming, 1930s.

TV Hulk Actor Lou Ferrigno gives thanks to Bragg Books. Lou went from puny to become Super Hulk! ➤

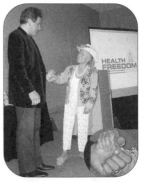

"I lost 102 lbs. with The Bragg Healthy Lifestyle and I have kept it off for over 15 years, staying away from white flour, sugar and other processed foods."
– Dee McCaffrey, Chemist & Diet Counselor, Tempe, AZ

Lou & Patricia in Chicago Health Freedom Expo.

PATRICIA CONTINUING BRAGG HEALTH CRUSADE!

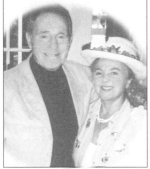

Jack LaLanne with Patricia.

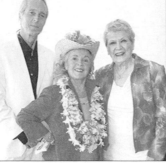

Jon & Elaine LaLanne with Patricia.

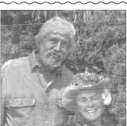

Patricia Bragg with Bill Galt inspired by Bragg Books, he founded Good Earth Restaurants.

Mother Nature Loves US!

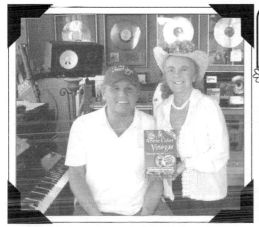

Patricia in studio with famous Beach Boy Bruce Johnston, Bragg follower over 40 years. He played for her their latest records.

Patricia with Jean-Michel Cousteau Ocean Explorer & Environmentalist. OceanFutures.org

Enjoy a Lifetime of Radiant Health

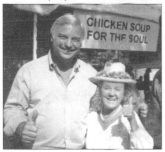

Patricia with Jack Canfield, Bragg follower, Motivational Speaker and Co-Producer of *Chicken Soup For The Soul.*

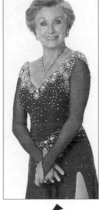

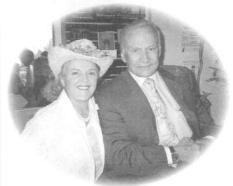

Patricia with Astronaut Buzz Aldrin, celebrating over 50 years since pilot of Apollo 11 first landed on the moon.

Famous Hollywood Actress Cloris Leachman, ardent health follower who sparkled with health and vitality said, *"Bragg Miracle of Fasting Book is a miracle . . . it cured my asthma, my years of arthritis and many other health problems. I praise Paul and Patricia daily for their Health Crusading!"*

PAUL & PATRICIA BRAGG
HEALTH CRUSADING

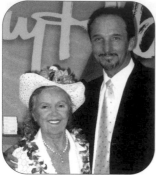

Patricia with Jay Robb.

Paul C. Bragg on the Merv Griffin Show, 1976.

Paul C. Bragg inspired me many years ago with the Miracle of Fasting Book and his pioneering philosophy on health. His daughter Patricia is a testament to the ageless value of living The Bragg Healthy Lifestyle. – Jay Robb, author of *The Fruit Flush*

During the many years Patricia worked with her father, she was right beside him, assisting him on Bragg Health Crusades worldwide. They were a great team, when you looked at them, you would see only two people headed in the same healthy direction!

I am a big fan of Paul C. Bragg. I fast and follow the Bragg Healthy Lifestyle daily. The world and I are blessed with the health teachings of Paul and Patricia Bragg!
– Tony Robbins • TonyRobbins.com

❀ **Dream big, think big and enjoy the many miracles.** ❀

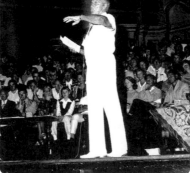

Paul – London Bragg Health Crusade.

Paul & Daughter Patricia, Royal Hawaiian, Honolulu.

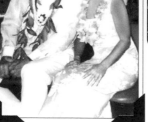

Actor Arthur Godfrey with Patricia, in Honolulu celebrating his 79th birthday.

Health Crusaders Paul C. Bragg and daughter Patricia traveled the world spreading health, inspiring millions to renew and revitalize their health.
Bragg Mottos:
3 John 2 and Genesis 6:3

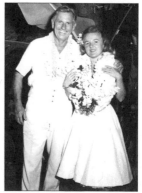

100 YEAR HISTORY OF BRAGG HEALTH BOOKS & PRODUCTS

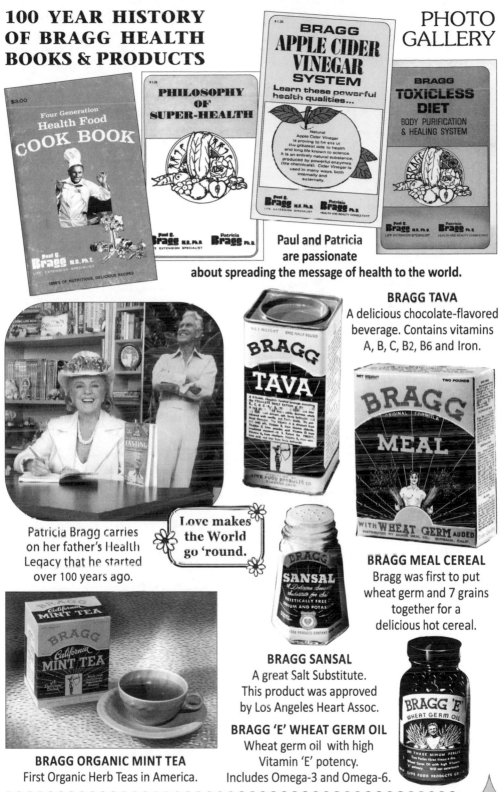

PHOTO GALLERY

$3.00

Four Generation
Health Food
COOK BOOK

Paul C. **Bragg** N.D. Ph.T.
LIFE EXTENSION SPECIALIST

1000'S OF NUTRITIOUS, DELICIOUS RECIPES

PHILOSOPHY OF SUPER-HEALTH

Paul C. **Bragg** N.D. Ph.T.
LIFE EXTENSION SPECIALIST

Patricia **Bragg** Ph.D.

#1.25

BRAGG APPLE CIDER VINEGAR SYSTEM

Learn these powerful health qualities...

Natural Apple Cider Vinegar is proving to be one of the greatest aids to health and long life known to science. It is an entirely natural substance, produced by powerful enzymes (life chemicals). Cider Vinegar is used in many ways, both internally and externally.

Paul C. **Bragg** N.D. Ph.D.
LIFE EXTENSION SPECIALIST

Patricia **Bragg** Ph.D.
HEALTH AND BEAUTY CONSULTANT

BRAGG TOXICLESS DIET
BODY PURIFICATION & HEALING SYSTEM

Paul C. **Bragg** N.D. Ph.D.
LIFE EXTENSION SPECIALIST

Patricia **Bragg** Ph.D.
HEALTH AND BEAUTY CONSULTANT

Paul and Patricia are passionate about spreading the message of health to the world.

Patricia Bragg carries on her father's Health Legacy that he started over 100 years ago.

Love makes the World go 'round.

BRAGG TAVA
A delicious chocolate-flavored beverage. Contains vitamins A, B, C, B2, B6 and Iron.

BRAGG **TAVA**
NET WEIGHT ONE HALF POUND

BRAGG **MEAL**
ORIGINAL FORMULA
NET WEIGHT TWO POUNDS
WITH **WHEAT GERM** ADDED

BRAGG MEAL CEREAL
Bragg was first to put wheat germ and 7 grains together for a delicious hot cereal.

BRAGG **SANSAL**

BRAGG ORGANIC MINT TEA
First Organic Herb Teas in America.

BRAGG SANSAL
A great Salt Substitute. This product was approved by Los Angeles Heart Assoc.

BRAGG 'E' WHEAT GERM OIL
Wheat germ oil with high Vitamin 'E' potency. Includes Omega-3 and Omega-6.

BRAGG **'E'**
WHEAT GERM OIL

"Our lives have completely turned around! Our family is feeling so healthy, we must tell you about it." – Gene & Joan Zollner, parents of 11, Washington

HALL of LEGENDS
Patricia Bragg

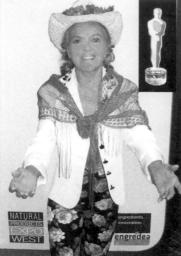

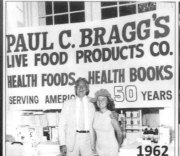

1962

Paul C. Bragg with Patricia, celebrating over 50 years of Bragg Health Products, Books & Crusading worldwide, spreading Health around the world.

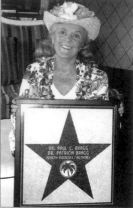

"Palm Spring Walk of Stars" – Patricia with Bragg Star.

Natural Foods Expo in Anaheim with 65,000 attendees from around the world honored Patricia Bragg and her father Paul C. Bragg as treasured Health Food Industry Legends.

BRAGG's 100th Anniversary Celebration

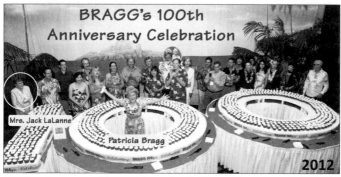

Mrs. Jack LaLanne

Patricia Bragg

2012

Patricia, Staff & 1,000 Friends celebrated our 100 years of Bragg Healthy Products, Books & Health Crusading! We are proud Pioneers in this Big Health Industry that is helping to keep the world healthier! With Blessings of Health, Peace & Love to You!

Patricia

100 Year Anniversary Party celebrated at the Natural Foods Expo in Anaheim

Bragg Hawaii Exercise Class

was founded by Worldwide Health Crusader and Fitness Legend, Dr. Paul C. Bragg. He wanted to create a dynamic, Free Community Exercise Class, and he often taught these classes himself for many years. Patricia Bragg continues her father's health legacy by supporting the Bragg Exercise Class and participates in the class whenever she is in Hawaii.

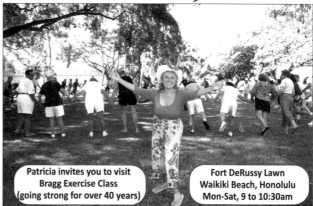

Patricia invites you to visit Bragg Exercise Class (going strong for over 40 years)

Fort DeRussy Lawn Waikiki Beach, Honolulu Mon-Sat, 9 to 10:30am

"Please make a record of your family history & background. Take pictures – make your own 'Photo Gallery.' Take videos – make movies of your children, spouse, mother and father, family gatherings, etc. These memories are precious & important to save for future generations." – Patricia Bragg

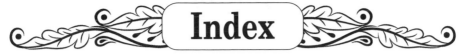

Index

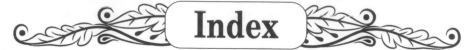

Index

A book is a garden, an orchard, a storehouse, a party, a mentor, a teacher, a guidepost, and a counsellor. – Henry Ward Beecher

All our dreams can come true – if we have the courage to pursue them. – Walt Disney

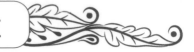

The Miracle of Fasting - Proven Throughout History

BY PAUL C. BRAGG, N.D., PH.D.
and PATRICIA BRAGG

In this newly revised best-seller, known to millions as the "bible of fasting" health pioneers and researchers Paul C. Bragg and Patricia Bragg teach why this ancient practice is key to health and energy, and critical to longevity and ageless vitality, due to our toxic environment and the stress of our daily lives. They share a detailed, step-by-step approach, accessible and informative for both beginners and experienced fasters. Our bodies must process not only our food and water, but the air we breathe, and whatever chemicals they may contain. Since detoxification and digestion take more energy than even strenuous athletic pursuits, fasting allows the mind and body to rest, renew and regenerate, to come into harmony and balance, and release the effects of stimulating foods like caffeine and sugars. The goal of fasting, say the authors, is to allow for the mind and body to self-heal. This concise, tightly edited *The Miracle of Fasting* is filled with personal stories of Paul C. Bragg's travels around the world, including a fasting journey in India with Mahatma Gandhi.

Healthy Heart - Learn the Facts

BY PAUL C. BRAGG, N.D., PH.D.
and PATRICIA BRAGG

Heart disease claims more American lives than any other illness and is the number one cause of death for women. World-renowned health pioneers Paul C. Bragg and Patricia Bragg teach time-tested, proven strategies for healing and maintaining a healthy heart for a long, active life! In a world filled with technological wizardry and products, the human heart still outperforms them all. That is – if that human heart is kept healthy. That is what the trailblazers Paul C. Bragg and Patricia Bragg have done in this book, sharing simple suggestions for lifestyle changes, nutritional support and exercises that will keep this most miraculous machine, your body, healthy and strong. You will learn how the heart works and how and why coronary disease is preventable and reversible. The authors provide an easy-to-follow blueprint for heart health that includes stress-release techniques, affirming that a positive mental outlook on life is a major element of heart health. The Braggs are legendary in the field of nutrition and health, and this newly revised and edited edition is a foundation of The Bragg Healthy Lifestyle. It is one of the most comprehensive heart health books on the market today.

Authored by America's First Family of Health
Live Longer – Healthier – Stronger Self-Improvement Library

Building Powerful Nerve Force & Positive Energy - Reduce Stress, Worry and Anger

BY PAUL C. BRAGG, N.D., PH.D.
and PATRICIA BRAGG

What is Nerve Force and why should you care about it? According to mental health trailblazers Paul C. Bragg and Patricia Bragg, "Nerve Force" is a type of life energy stored in the nerves, muscles, organs, and brain. The more Nerve Force you have, the quicker you can re-charge it, and the healthier, happier, and more satisfying a life you will lead. If you suffer from burnout, stress, fatigue, anxiety, insomnia or depression, this book is for you! We know that the ability to feel joy and peace is essential to a complete experience of vitality and wellness. Our thoughts, our attitudes, our outlook, and our emotional well-being are all dependent on having a powerful "Nerve Force." Just like any muscle that we can develop and strengthen, we can build our Nerve Force so that we are resilient, relaxed, and calm, even during times of stress. Paul C. Bragg and Patricia Bragg show you how with simple mental exercises and suggestions for specific foods that replenish your Nerve Force, as well as foods that deplete it, in this newly revised edition of *Building Powerful Nerve Force & Positive Energy* the father-daughter team explains to readers the reward of paying attention to the energy that is responsible for not only our physical capabilities and our vital body functions, but our ability to process information and feel centered and grounded, no matter what life throws at us. They teach us that maintaining a healthy Nerve Force, leads to a balanced and fruitful life.

Super Power Breathing - For Optimum Health & Healing

BY PAUL C. BRAGG, N.D., PH.D.
and PATRICIA BRAGG

Do you sometimes find that you are panting instead of breathing? Many of us do! This can cause headaches, anxiety, fatigue, and brain fog. The quality of our breath determines the quality of our life! This book teaches us how to breathe in a way that replenishes the body with the oxygen it so deeply craves. "The more effectively we breathe, the more effectively we live," write the authors, world-renowned health pioneers Paul C. Bragg and Patricia Bragg. "Super Power Breathing can make your life-force stronger, calmer and smarter." The Super Power Breathing program has been followed by Olympic athletes and millions of Bragg followers, and is filled with simple exercises for energizing and rejuvenating your breath, and your whole body. Research shows that we use only one-fourth to one-half of our lung capacity with each breath. This starves our body much like if we are depriving it of food. We are slowly robbing our body of its most vital, invisible nourishment – oxygen. In its newly revised form, the Bragg Super Power Breathing Program will give you all the tools you need to shift from shallow breathing to taking deep, oxygen-filled, life-giving breaths!

Water - The Shocking Truth

BY PAUL C. BRAGG, N.D., PH.D.
and PATRICIA BRAGG

The water you drink can literally make or break your health. The purity of our water is the most critical element in maintaining radical vitality, and healing from illness and disease. In this newly revised edition of *Water: The Shocking Truth*, health crusaders Paul C. Bragg and Patricia Bragg reveal the dangers of tap water, which research shows can be responsible for many ailments, due to the addition of dangerous chemicals such as fluoride and chlorine. In this book, the trailblazing father-daughter team teach the many functions water performs in the body, from regulating the various systems to flushing the body of waste and toxins. But what if the substance we use to cleanse our bodies is itself polluted? With the mandatory fluoridation of water in the municipal water systems, the authors assert that has been the case for decades. Added to the public water supply to prevent tooth decay starting in the 1950s, fluoride has long been known to be a toxin, used in pesticides and rat poisons. Learn what types of water are optimal to drink, how and why to detox your body with nature's most life-giving liquid, and the health-and-life-saving value of installing a water filter in your shower!

Bragg Back & Foot Fitness Program -
Keys to a Pain-Free Back & Strong Healthy Feet

BY PAUL C. BRAGG, N.D., PH.D.
and PATRICIA BRAGG

If you are suffering with back or foot pain, look no further for a comprehensive program that will restore health to the parts of your body that carry you through life! Remember when we were children, and we had the kind of energy and flexibility to play for hours? Agile and active, we could twist, bend, stretch and climb with little effort. However, hours looking at a computer screen, a sedentary lifestyle and poor posture can take their toll. Eventually our backs start to hurt and cramp with every movement, and our feet ache after just a short walk. We start feeling "old." In *Bragg Back & Foot Fitness Program*, the father-daughter team of world-renowned health pioneers, Paul C. Bragg and Patricia Bragg teach how to speed the healing of injuries and develop a strong and flexible back and healthy feet, rejuvenating and re-energizing our bodies in the process. The trailblazing health experts who brought wellness and vitality to millions, including fitness guru Jack LaLanne, outline the keys to a healthy spine, pain-free back and bunion-free feet through nutritional support and clearly illustrated, simple exercises, as well as other tips for posture and massage. Paul and Patricia Bragg reveal the healing properties of herbs, effective ways to practice foot reflexology, how to deal with arthritis, athlete's foot, plantar fasciitis, and foot problems caused by diabetes. By following the authors' Back and Foot Care Program, you can begin to treat your body as Mother Nature intended you to, and creating painless feet, a strong back and a powerful body will begin!

PATRICIA BRAGG
Health Crusader and "Angel of Health and Healing"

Author, Lecturer, Nutritionist, Health & Lifestyle Educator to World Leaders, Hollywood Stars, Singers, Athletes & Millions.

Patricia is a life-long health advocate and activist, admired internationally for her passionate work promoting healthy living. For many years she traveled the world, teaching The Bragg Healthy Lifestyle for physical, spiritual, emotional health and joy. She was invited to give lectures, visited radio shows, was profiled in magazines and appealed to people of all ages, nationalities and walks-of-life. Together with Paul, she co-authored a collection of ten books, with inspiration and techniques for living a long, vital, happy life. Now in her 90s and living on an organic farm in California, Patricia herself is a testament to these teachings and the sparkling symbol of health, perpetual youth and radiant energy.

PAUL C. BRAGG, N.D., Ph.D.
Life Extension Specialist • World Health Crusader
Lecturer and Advisor to Olympic Athletes, Royalty, Stars & Millions.
Originator of Health Food Stores & Founder of Health Movement Worldwide

Paul C. Bragg was at the forefront of the modern health movement, having inspired generations to turn toward wellness. At a young age, Paul turned his own health around by developing an eating, breathing and exercise program to build strength and vitality. From this life-changing experience, he pledged to dedicate the rest of his life to promoting a healthy lifestyle. He opened one of the country's first health food stores, which eventually led to the creation of the Bragg Live Foods company. With a devoted following, Paul traveled giving lectures and sharing his expertise, while serving as an advisor to athletes and movie stars alike. Even Jack LaLanne, the original television fitness guru, credited Paul with having introduced him to the importance of healthy living. In addition to the books Paul wrote with Patricia, they co-hosted television and radio shows and worked together to bring wellness to the world. Paul himself excelled in athletics, loved the ocean and the outdoors, and radiated with health and a warm smile.

Patricia inspires you to Renew, Rejuvenate and Revitalize your Life with "The Bragg Healthy Lifestyle" Books. Millions have benefitted from these life-changing philosophies with a longer, healthier, happier life!

Take Time for 12 Things

1. Take time to **Work** –
   it is the price of success.
2. Take time to **Think** –
   it is the source of power.
3. Take time to **Play** –
   it is the secret of youth.
4. Take time to **Read** –
   it is the foundation of knowledge.
5. Take time to **Worship** –
   it is the highway of reverence and
   washes the dust of earth from our eyes.
6. Take time to **Help and Enjoy Friends** –
   it is the source of happiness.
7. Take time to **Love and Share** –
   it is the one sacrament of life.
8. Take time to **Dream** –
   it hitches the soul to the stars.
9. Take time to **Laugh** –
   it is the singing that helps life's loads.
10. Take time for **Beauty** –
    it is everywhere in nature.
11. Take time for **Health** –
    it is the true wealth and treasure of life.
12. Take time to **Plan** –
    it is the secret of being able to have time
    for the first 11 things.

YOUR BIRTHRIGHT

HEALTH

CULTIVATE IT

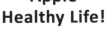

**Have an
Apple
Healthy Life!**

3 John 2

154

*Teach me thy way, LORD, lead me in a straight path,
because of my oppressors. – Psalm 27:11*